Animal Diseases

Control and Treatment

Animal Diseases
Control and Treatment

Neil Turner

Editor

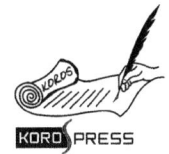

KOROS PRESS LIMITED
London, UK

Animal Diseases: Control and Treatment

© 2012
Printed in 2017 for Sale in the Indian Subcontinent

Published by
Koros Press Limited
3 The Pines, Rubery B45 9FF, Rednal,
Birmingham, United Kingdom

Tel.: +44-7826-930152
Email: info@korospress.com
www.korospress.com

ISBN: 978-1-78163-125-6
Editor: Neil Turner

Printed in UK

British Library Cataloguing in Publication Data
A CIP record for this book is available from the British Library

10 9 8 7 6 5 4 3 2 1

Contents

Preface

The health of swine can best be ensured by a combination of prevention and treatment of diseases. Prevention includes both biosecurity and vaccination. Biosecurity includes isolating pigs from other species, both domestic and feral, as well as isolating pigs from each other by age. A major health risk is the introduction of new pigs into a resident population, because pigs brought from other farms are likely to carry disease-causing organisms to which the resident population has not developed any immunity. Human visitors also pose some risk, which can be mitigated by having them put on clean clothes and boots at a swine facility. A strict sanitation and traffic control program minimizes opportunities for new disease organisms to enter the herd, while systematic vaccination reduces the likelihood of routine diseases. A comprehensive herd health program also includes optimum nutrition, comfortable housing, excellent ventilation, and vigorous parasite control. Safe and effective vaccines are available for many swine diseases, and producers work with their veterinarians to develop health programs that will alleviate infections of diseases prevalent in their local areas. Antibiotics may be added to the feed or water or be given by injection. Low-level doses of antibiotics, known as subtherapeutic, in the feed assist in preventing various bacteria from expressing disease symptoms.

Infected pigs exhibiting disease symptoms may be treated with therapeutic levels. Producers treating pigs with any medication must be aware of and follow minimum withdrawal periods before the pigs are marketed. Improvements in breeding, disease control, management, and feed formulation have all contributed to faster gains and lower feed requirements per kilogram of weight gain. The use of antibiotics began in the early 1950s in the United States, and the practice immediately resulted in increasing the rate of weight gain in nursery pigs (especially in regions with less favourable sanitation) by as much as 20 percent and by about 5 percent in pigs weighing more than 50 kg (110 pounds). Antibiotics became a standard ingredient in most young pigs' diets. Nevertheless, many European countries have restricted subtherapeutic use of antibiotics for growth promotion in livestock diets because of concern that antibiotic-resistant bacteria that infect humans may develop. Pigs are subject to many infectious and parasitic diseases. Diseases can be divided into infectious and noninfectious. Infectious diseases are transmitted between animals and include various bacterial, viral, and mycoplasmal organisms, as well as parasites. Noninfectious diseases include poisonous plants, toxins, nutritional excesses and deficiencies, and metabolic diseases such as ulcers.

Common diseases controllable by vaccination include transmissible gastroenteritis, which is often fatal to piglets (even when vaccinated); leptospirosis, which can also infect humans and most warm-blooded animals; pseudorabies, a viral disease that causes high mortality in piglets; and erysipelas, a bacterial infection that causes inflammation of the skin and swelling and stiffness of the joints. Cholera and foot-and-mouth disease, formerly controlled by vaccination, are now usually controlled by slaughter of infected herds. Necrotic enteritis and other infections of the intestinal tract are largely controlled by antibiotics. Atrophic rhinitis produces sneezing, crooked snouts, and poor performance and is controlled by a combination of vaccination and antibiotics. Parasitic diseases can be divided into external and internal parasites. External parasites include lice and mites (which cause mange). Effective topical and internal preparations are available for their control or elimination. Internal parasites include various worms, which can be controlled through effective treatment with anthelmintics and through improvements in sanitation. Internal parasites are less of a problem when pigs are raised on slatted floors, which reduce spreading and re-infection by separating the pigs from their manure and other intermediary parasite hosts.

The present book has been carefully compiled and edited to meet the long felt needs of increasingly number of students and researchers who have to deal with the different aspects of animal diseases.

—Editor

Chapter 1

The Effect of Natural Toxins on Reproduction in Livestock

Reproductive efficiency is the most important economic factor in livestock production. Thus, the hypothalamo-pituitary-gonadal regulatory axis, accessory sexual organ functionality, and the complex events involved in fertilization, implantation, and embryonic and fetal development may be sensitive to therapeutic agents, environmental pollutants, and natural toxicants. There are many factors that adversely affect reproduction, one of which is toxic substances in the diets of animals. Toxic materials can affect reproductive success by causing abortions, interfering with libido, estrus, oogenesis, or spermatogenesis, causing emaciation and subsequent abnormal mating behaviour, birth defects, and increasing the time between parturition and rebreeding.

Examples of natural toxicants in poisonous plants interfering with reproduction are numerous. Abortion in livestock from locoweeds, ponderosa pine needles, broom snakeweeds, fescue, and others are reported in studies. Selenium and seleniferous forage inhibit estrus in cattle and swine. Emaciation and temporary illness from sneezeweeds, bitterweed, locoweed, larkspur, lupines, and others may interfere with mating. Embryonic loss and birth defects from Veratrum, lupines, locoweeds, poison hemlock, and so on, may occur. As suggested, toxins have many diverse and economically adverse effects on reproductive performance in livestock.

Colostrum for the Dairy Calf

The cost of raising replacement dairy animals increases if calf-rearing results in higher-than-normal mortality or requires medicine to treat preventable diseases.

At birth, a calf has a poorly developed immune system. The placenta does not allow the transfer of antibodies, also known as immunoglobulins (Ig), from the mother to the fetus during pregnancy.

True colostrum is the "first milk", which is rich with the antibodies that provide the calf protection from diseases in early life until the calf's own immune system becomes functional. Colostrum is also important as the first source of nutrients after birth.

Antibodies are proteins that identify and destroy disease-causing organisms, or pathogens, in the calf. Three major types of Ig (G, M and A) are typically found in the colostrum of dairy cows in percentages of 85%-90%, 5%-10% and 5%-10%, respectively.

The three types of immunoglobulins have specific roles in the immune system. The primary role of IgG is to identify and help destroy invading pathogens. IgG can move out of the bloodstream and into other areas of the body where it helps identify pathogens. The principal role of IgM is to identify and destroy bacteria that have entered the blood. IgA attaches to the membranes that line many organs, such as the intestine, and prevents pathogens from attaching and causing disease.

Timing

Timing is critical to a successful colostrum-feeding management program. The ability of a calf's small intestine to absorb immunoglobulins drops rapidly over the first few hours of life. By 24 hr of age, the ability to absorb immunoglobulins is nearly nonexistent. If a calf has not received any colostrum within 12 hr of birth, it is unlikely to be able to absorb enough antibodies to have adequate immunity. For this reason, a calf should receive the first feeding of colostrum within 1 hr of birth when possible.

Passive immunity is the temporary protection that the calf receives from the cow through the transfer of maternal antibodies present in colostrum. Passive immunity protects the calf until its own immune system becomes active. With active immunity, an older calf is mature enough to produce antibodies in response to vaccinations or to fight infections that it is exposed to.

The goal for proper colostrum feeding is for the calf to achieve a minimum blood serum IgG level greater than 10 mg/mL. As an alternative to testing for serum IgG levels, serum total protein levels may be measured. A serum total protein level of 5.2 g/dL is considered equivalent to the serum IgG level of 10 mg/mL.

"Failure of passive transfer" (FPT) occurs when the acceptable levels of total protein or IgG are not achieved by 24-48 hr after birth. Canadian and American reports often show that as many as 35%-40%

of dairy calves suffer from FTP, which indicates that many calves have inadequate immunity and are more likely to get sick. A recent study reported serum total protein levels in Ontario dairy calves; approximately 35% of calves had FPT.

It is accepted that the higher the concentration of IgG or serum total protein levels in the calf 48 hr after birth, the greater the protection the calf has against disease pathogens.

A study by the U.S. National Animal Health Monitoring System found that calves with low immunoglobulin levels in their blood 2 days after birth had a death rate over the next 8 weeks that was more than twice that of calves with acceptable levels of serum immunoglobulins.

Quantity

The best practice is to feed 4 L of high-quality colostrum to Holstein calves within 1 hr of birth. A second feeding of 2?3 L of colostrum should be given within the next 8 hr. Calves that are bottle-fed colostrum have a better chance of receiving enough immunoglobulins than calves left to nurse from their mother. Calves that fail to drink on their own within 3 hr of birth should be given colostrum by esophageal feeder.

Quality

The immunoglobulin content in the first "milking" colostrum is typically 5%-6% (50-60 g/L), but can range from less than 2% (20 g/L) to greater than 15% (150 g/L).

The concentration of antibodies in colostrum decreases rapidly with each milking as the transition from colostrum to milk production occurs. Usually, the second milking has 65% as much immunoglobulins as the first milking. By the third milking, the level has fallen to 40% of the first milking. Some differences in the composition between true colostrum, transitional milk and whole milk are shown in Table.

Nutrients in colostrum, such as fat and protein, are also important to the calf for growth and development. The lactose concentration in colostrum is less than is present in whole milk, which reduces the chance of diarrhea in the newborn calf.

Dairy breeds produce lower concentrations of immunoglobulins in their colostrum than beef breeds. Among the common dairy breeds, Holsteins tend to have the lowest level and Jerseys the highest.

First-lactation heifers usually have lower levels than older cows that are in their third or greater lactation. Cows that have had less than a 4-week dry period usually have lower levels of antibodies.

Cleanliness

A significant challenge of colostrum feeding is keeping it clean. While feeding colostrum is essential to provide passive immunity for the calf, it is also one of the first ways to potentially expose the calf to such pathogens as *E. coli, Salmonella* or *Mycobacterium avium paratuberculosis*, the bacterial species responsible for Johne's disease. Pathogens can also cause diseases such as scours and septicemia and may interfere with passive absorption of the antibodies from the gut into the circulation system. Clean udders, milking equipment and calf-feeding equipment well before harvesting, storing and feeding colostrum.

Feed calves colostrum that has a total bacteria count of less than 100,000 colony-forming units (CFU)/mL and a total coliform count of less than 10,000 CFU/mL.

An Ontario study in 2002 found that 12% of colostrum samples had high levels of bacteria. The study concluded that the source of the bacteria was from either a dirty udder or dirty collection container. Similarly, results from a recent U.S. study reported bacterial results from the colostrum on 12 dairy farms. In that study, the average total plate count was 16.1 million CFU/mL, and the total coliform count was 2.7 million CFU/mL, indicating that dairy farmers should pay more attention to colostrum cleanliness.

Storage

Colostrum can be refrigerated cold at 1°C-2°C (33°F-35°F) for up to a week or kept frozen at -20°C (-4°F) for up to year. Avoid frost-free freezers. Two-litre plastic containers or freezer bags are ideal. If using freezer bags, double-bag the colostrum.

Thaw the colostrum in 50°C (120°F) water. Do not thaw at room temperature, as bacteria double every 20-30 min. at room temperature.

Colostrum can also be thawed in a microwave, with care. Microwave the colostrum on low for short periods of time. Avoid hot spots and mix partially thawed containers if necessary.

Recent research at the University of Minnesota found that colostrum can be heated to 60°C (140°F) without damaging the antibodies. However, when the colostrum was heated to 63°C (145°F), the antibodies were reduced by 34%.

Do not mix colostrum from two or more cows.

Colostrum can also be pasteurised on farm to reduce the presence of pathogens. The newer pasteurisation equipment is convenient to use. It can provide a very effective method of reducing pathogens to improve colostrum cleanliness and dramatically reduce the potential for diseases to be transmitted by feeding colostrum. It is important to keep pasteurisation equipment clean and to follow manufacturers?

directions for both temperature and time of treatment so as not to destroy the antibodies present in the colostrum. Pasteurising colostrum significantly reduces the level of bacteria present. However, to reduce bacterial regrowth, pasteurised colostrum must be properly stored, as described above, until it is fed.

As a final alternative, if sufficient amounts of high-quality colostrum are not available, commercial colostrum supplements can be a valuable tool for increasing calf immunity or for use as a disease-management strategy when transmission of disease from the mother to the calf is an issue.

In the U.S., some colostrum supplements use bovine serum as the source of immunoglobulins. These products have not been approved in Canada, and their ability to achieve satisfactory immune status in dairy calves is debatable. Maternal colostrum replacement products prepared from colostrum from healthy cows are available in Canada, and published research supports its effectiveness at increasing immunity protection in dairy calves.

Follow manufacturer's directions with these products.

Testing

Testing equipment can be purchased from a number of farm suppliers.

A colostrum hydrometre, often called a Colostrometre®, estimates the immunoglobulins in the colostrum by measuring the specific gravity of colostrum. Accurate measurements require that the temperature of the colostrum be correct, typically, at room temperature. Higher or lower temperatures result in incorrect readings. Follow manufacturer's directions. Some manufacturers provide information to adjust readings if tested at other temperatures.

Readings of more than 50 g/L for colostrum IgG concentrations are desirable.

Refractometres are commonly used by veterinarians to evaluate the degree of passive transfer in calves. Refractometres are used to estimate the total serum protein level in the calf. Readings of 5.2 g/dL or greater indicate successful passive transfer.

Summary

Colostrum is the critical first step to the health and survival of newborn calves. The successful transfer of the antibody protection in colostrum from cow to calf is based on four key factors:

- How quickly the calf receives colostrum after birth - within 1 hr is best.
- How much colostrum the calf receives - 4 L at first feeding.
- The immunoglobulin concentration in the colostrum.

Sanitation for Fly and Disease Management at Confined Livestock Facilities

Flies

The stable fly and house fly are the major insect pests at confined livestock units. The stable fly has a piercing-type mouthpart which is used to pierce the skin to obtain a blood meal. House flies do not bite because they have a sponging-type mouthpart with which they feed on semi-liquid material. The life cycles of the two species are similar, consisting of eggs, larvae (maggots), pupae, and the adult. During summer months the stable fly completes its life cycle in about three weeks and the house fly in about two weeks. Both species deposit eggs in wet, decaying organic matter. This includes spilled livestock feed and manure mixed with soil and moisture. In addition, the house fly will breed in fresh manure. The two species generally overwinter as slowly developing larvae in breeding areas below the frost line. The house fly may breed during the winter in warm buildings if breeding material is present.

Cattle under attack by stable flies will bunch together with each animal attempting to find a position within the bunch which protects their front legs—the favoured feeding site of the flies. Considerable energy is expended by foot stomping, tail switching, and throwing the head down toward the front legs in an effort to dislodge the flies or prevent feeding.

Stable flies reduce weight gains, milk production, and feed efficiency—both from their feeding and because of the bunching behaviour of cattle which may induce or increase heat stress.

House flies have not been shown to reduce animal weight gain and feed efficiency but are known to transmit several animal diseases. The disease organisms recovered from house flies range from viruses to nematodes. The most common of these are the bacteria associated with enteric infections. The house fly mouthparts and feeding habits (filth sources) make it efficient in transmitting bacterial and viral agents. Over 100 different disease organisms have been recovered from house flies, and the fly has been implicated in the transmission of 65 of these. Transmission may simply involve the mechanical transfer of the disease agent from the mouthparts or body of the fly to the animal host. In other cases, the disease agent may multiply in the fly and be transmitted after populations of the disease agent build up to high numbers or it changes to a different life stage.

Stable flies, because of their blood-feeding habits, have also been suspected of transmitting diseases, but most research in disease transmission studies with the stable fly have proven negative. Mastitis in dairy herds is one of the exceptions. The mastitis organisms are routinely spread by the stable fly to the teat ends of heifers or lactating cows. Mastitis, the most costly disease of dairy cattle, is caused when the bacteria invade the teat and gain entrance to the mammary gland.

One other important economic factor associated with stable flies and house flies is the threat of nuisance lawsuits. Generally odour, dust, and flies are cited together as constituting a nuisance by the plaintiffs. The lawsuit may seek damages or, perhaps worse, request closing of the livestock facility.

Effective house fly and stable fly control cannot be achieved with insecticides alone. Proper animal manure management and sanitation must be the major element in a good fly control program. Confined livestock facilities should be designed or modified to facilitate ease in cleaning and to minimise accumulations of manure, spilled feed and other sources of organic debris.

Breeding Areas

In feedlots, major fly breeding areas include: 1) fence lines where manure mixed with wet soil accumulates; 2) along feeding aprons where, because of the slope of the aprons, moisture and manure accumulate; 3) at the edges of potholes, in pen corners, and around gates; 4) along pen drainage channels or edges of holding ponds at the water-soil interface unless it is sloped enough to drain and dry quickly; 5) along the sloping edges of mounds where moisture runoff occurs; 6) around waterers if leakage or spillage occurs; 7) at the edge of and under feed bunks; 8) in and around feed handling facilities if the feed becomes wet; 9) at the edges of stored manure, if the edges are loosely packed and wet; and 10) at the edge of silage and haylage.

In addition, excessive moisture may provide fly-breeding areas under round bales in and around old hay or straw stack butts and in sick pens and horse stables if hay or straw bedding is used.

Fly breeding areas at dairies might include any of the areas described for feedlots, but fly breeding might also occur under and around self-feeding forage racks and in calf hutches or pens where hay or straw bedding is used.

Fly breeding at swine units is restricted primarily to the house fly. Stable flies will breed in wet, spilled feed around swine units but are rarely, if ever, found breeding in wet soil-swine manure mixtures as is the house fly. The most common fly breeding areas will differ to some extent with the type of facility but basically occur at any location where swine manure or wet feed stuffs are allowed to remain for a period of 10-14 days. In swine confinement buildings, where manure is collected below the slatted floor pens, a crust occasionally occurs unless some type of agitation is provided.

House flies may breed in the crust just below the surface. Agitation provided by the manure dropping from the slatted floor will suffice if enough liquid is available and the depth of the drop is greater than one foot. Manure may also accumulate in the upper corners just below the slatted floors. The same situation is true for cattle confinement buildings.

In modified open front or open lots, the main fly breeding areas may be under and around the self-feeders or in the corners of the facility. While the accumulation of the manure or spilled feed may be relatively small, an area about a square yard in size will allow several thousand flies to develop in a period of two to three weeks.

Fly Management

Reduction of fly breeding areas in feedlots is dependent primarily on manure management and keeping the lots dry. Mounds are a key element in this process. They should be built and maintained to provide a dry area for the cattle and drainage for the excess moisture to move from the pens to the drainage system. During wet periods, the wet edges of the mounds can be scraped into the lot in a thin layer to facilitate rapid drying.

Maximum stocking rates create tramping action that helps in drying. The lots also can be dragged periodically which helps maintain a dry surface. The area behind the feeding apron should be scraped at two week intervals and the manure either removed or spread out in the lot for rapid drying. Drainage systems should be maintained with enough slope to move the moisture to the holding ponds rapidly which allows for rapid drying as well.

Haylage and silage piles may have drainage at the edges. The seepage provides an excellent fly-breeding site. Covering this seepage area with black plastic should create enough heat to kill the developing fly larvae. If manure is used as fertilizer and spread directly on farm fields, care should be taken to spread the manure thin enough for rapid drying. If the manure is spread at depths of three to four inches or more and enough moisture is present, it may allow fly breeding.

Water tanks should be surrounded by a concrete apron and equipped with a drain line to facilitate cleaning without creating a muddy area in the lot. Float valves on waterers should be protected to prevent animals from causing an overflow. Livestock pens usually have enough organic matter present to create a fly breeding area wherever water accumulates.

Feedlots designed or modified to meet the Environmental Protection Agency?s pollution runoff standards can have an additional fly breeding area in the debris basin. The purpose of the debris basin is to intercept the feedlot runoff, allow the solids to settle and channel the liquids into the holding pond. The basin should be sloped enough to prevent water from standing and provide quick drying. Solids should be removed regularly to prevent fly breeding.

If spray mists are used to cool cattle or hogs or to settle dust, care should be taken to prevent puddles from forming. Dragging the surface of the lot may fill in low areas where puddles form.

Each livestock unit is different and there may be fly breeding occurring in only two or three locations. However, since even small amounts of fly-breeding material can support large numbers of flies, these areas should be located and removed. Manure management and sanitation can be expensive but should be considered a required management practice in livestock production. The benefits (better animal performance, more efficient use of insecticides, better working conditions for employees, more attractive facility for commercial customers, reduced risk of nuisance lawsuits, and reduced chances of disease outbreaks) may offset the expense.

Accurate Detection of Bruising Improves Carcase Value & Welfare

Females and older animals are more susceptible to bruising at slaughter and more accurate detection methods may identify who is economically responsible for losses in carcase value due to bruising. There are a number of external causes of bruises that are sustained during the last hours and days before beef animals are slaughtered and animal factors, such as sex and age, may contribute to the development of bruises, at least in some cases. Just some of the findings of a review by Dutch and Chilean scientists, led by Wageningen University's Ana Strappini.

"Better understanding is still needed of the biological mechanisms accounting for the higher bruise rates in females and older animals," she said, adding that it was also clear that beef cattle sold through markets can suffer bruising that could have been avoided by transporting animals directly from the farm to the slaughterhouse.

Studies of bruises, as detected on carcases at the slaughterhouse, may provide useful information about the traumatic situations the animals endure during the pre-slaughter period.

Many aspects of cattle transport contribute to bruising. Transport conditions, such as stocking density and duration of the journey, seem to have more effect on bruising than distance travelled. "But finding an optimal stocking density for livestock transport under different conditions is still a contentious issue," said Dr Strappini.

"Bruised tissues may store historical information about the harmful situations that the animal underwent prior to slaughter. The farmer and the transport companies have economic incentives to prevent and reduce bruising. However, slaughterhouses do not have simple and accurate methods for post-mortem age estimation of bruises to assess accurately when bruises were sustained.

This is a relevant problem, due to the importance of having to decide who is economically accountable for the losses. Although the number of bruises, their anatomical location, severity and even the healing process might offer a rapid tool for identifying and evaluating the circumstances during the pre-slaughter period such as high stocking density, rough handling or inappropriate facility infrastructure, other sensitive techniques should be considered for refined assessments of the time the bruises were incurred."

"More investigation of the time between bruising and slaughter may help to clarify the risk factors that have contributed to the occurrence of bruises and will also help to identify the risks for animal welfare," she added.

The modern diagnostic techniques applied when evaluating human bruises may be studied for bovine bruises as well. "Immunohistochemistry and cytochemistry seem to be promising methods to be applied to measure morphological or biochemical changes, which can clearly be distinguished from non-bruised tissues."

"But age assessment of bruises continues to be a crude process. A wide variety of factors intrinsic to the animal can influence the inflammatory process and subsequent repair.

"Normal biological variation among animals is therefore bound to result in substantial overlap among proposed time frames in the healing process."

Greenhouse Gases and Environmental Impacts of the Livestock Industry

We have a severe effect on grazing land and livestock production systems Pierre Gerber, Livestock Policy Officer Animal Production and Health Division at the FAO, told the recent World Meat Congress in Cape Town, South Africa.

He said it is a great challenge for food security and the security of the public's health and biodiversity and it is also a challenge for the livestock industry.

Dr Gerber said that at present 3.4 billion hectares around the world is devoted to pasture land - 26 per cent of the total of "emerged lands". While this was being used to a low intensity in the developing nations, the intensity of production was increasing in the Latin American countries.

A large part of this pasture land is too dry or too cold for crop use, and only sparsely inhabited.

While the grazing area is not increasing on a global scale, in tropical Latin America there is rapid expansion of pastures, which is encroaching into valuable ecosystems, with 0.3 to 0.4 per cent of forest lost to pasture annually, Dr Gerber said.

Ranching is a primary reason for this deforestation. About 20 per cent of the world's pastures and rangeland have been degraded to some extent - maybe as much as 73 per cent in dry areas.

This growing intensity of production is reflected in the fact that global production of meat is expected to more than double form 229 million tonnes in 1999/2001 to 465 million tonnes by 2050 and milk production in the same period will go up from 580 million tonnes to 1,043 million tonnes.

The bulk of this growth will be in the developing countries - Brazil, China, India and Russia in particular.

At the same time the global demand for livestock products is also expected to double.

The total area dedicated to feed crop production is 471 million hectares, equivalent to 33 per cent of the total arable land and most of this is in the developed countries.

Recent reports from the UN and other organisations show that land use changes that have followed deforestation contribute 18.3 per cent to total greenhouse gas emissions, while agriculture accounts for 13.5 per cent (six per cent of which is agricultural soils and 5.1 per cent is livestock and manure) and the transportation sector accounts for 13.5 per cent with 10 per cent down to road transport.

Dr Gerber said that estimates of greenhouse gas emissions for the livestock sector are substantial when the different forms of emissions throughout the livestock commodity chain are taken into account.

Emissions come from feed production, such as chemical fertilizer production, deforestation for pasture and feed crops, cultivation of feed crops, feed transport and soil organic matter losses in pastures and feed crops. The emissions also come from animal production, such as enteric fermentation and methane and nitrous oxide emissions from manure and as a result of the transportation of animal products.

Dr Gerber said that livestock production contributes about nine per cent of the total carbon dioxide emissions produced by human activity, but 37 per cent of methane and 65 per cent of nitrous oxide emissions.

In total there are 7.1 billion tonnes of CO_2 produced through feed and livestock production in the world and he said that CO_2 releases resulting from fossil fuel consumption used for the production of feed grains (tractors, fertilizer production, drying, milling and transporting) and feed oil crops also need to be attributed to livestock.

The same applies to the processing and transport of animal products.

Relative Greenhouse Gas Contributions Along the Food Chain

Dr Gerber told the conference that there is a similar impact from the livestock sector on water usage throughout the world.

The livestock sector accounts for about eight per cent of the total water used and most of this is used on feed crops and irrigation of pasture land.

There are also consequences for the water supply through the pollution of water by manure and pathogens and contaminants from livestock and freed production and there are consequences for the erosion of the soil through grazing animals and intensive rearing of animals.

The growing intensity of livestock production is changing the biodiversity of the world and is having an effect of different ecosystems.

"Climate change is a big problem, but there are other issues as well," Dr Gerber said.

He said the industry and governments need to control land use and control the carbon and nitrogen in cultivated soil. He said it is necessary to manage livestock production better for productivity gain and also for manure management.

He added that given the projected expansion of the livestock sector, major corrective measures need to be taken to address the environmental impact of livestock production, which will otherwise worsen dramatically.

Growing economies and populations, together with the increasing scarcity of environmental resources and rising environmental problems, are more and more demanding enhanced environmental services, such as clean air and water, and recreation areas.

He said that while there will be an increasing intensification in livestock production, the challenge will be to make the process environmentally acceptable.

With extensive land-based production the decision makers will have to ensure that it includes environmental parameters particularly in vulnerable areas.

Dr Gerber added that policy makers need to provide a framework for landscape maintenance, biodiversity protection, clean water and eventually carbon sequestration from extensive grazing systems, in addition to that for the production of conventional livestock commodities.

"Policy decisions have to take into account environmental and health aspects of livestock production," he said.

"And the FAO is endeavouring to raise awareness of these problems."

A strong political will and urgency, together with the identification of potential contributors and beneficiaries, are required to initiate action and investment, Dr Gerber concluded.

Plant-Produced Protein Eases Dairy Cow Infection

Coliform mastitis is the most prevalent form of clinical mastitis in the dairy industry and is mainly caused by the *Escherichia coli* bacterium. Use of antibiotics to control mastitis infections can be expensive and carries with it concerns about the emergence of antibiotic-resistant bacteria. Yet mastitis is expensive too, costing dairy farmers an estimated $2 billion annually from incapacitated cows and milk that can't be sold.

Now, ARS molecular biologist Lev Nemchinov and plant pathologist Rosemarie Hammond have endowed a potato virus with a gene that— when introduced into a host plant—prompts the plant to produce a therapeutic protein called "CD14." First isolated by Dante Zarlenga of the ARS Bovine Functional Genomics Laboratory, this beneficial protein can be extracted from the plant and used to treat mastitis.

Nemchinov and Hammond are with the Molecular Plant Pathology Laboratory at Beltsville, Maryland. Their engineered, or recombinant, virus is called "PVX/CD14," for "potato virus X carrying the gene of therapeutic protein CD14."

Protein Power

The researchers extracted enough CD14 protein from the inoculated plants for field tests. Their colleagues, dairy scientist Max Paape and microbiologist Douglas Bannerman with the ARS Bovine Functional Genomics Laboratory, Beltsville, Maryland, tested the purified protein's ability to alleviate mastitis in dairy cows.

CD14 is known to help the immune system fight infection, but it is present in the cow's mammary gland at low levels. CD14 binds to a molecule known as "lipopolysaccharide," located on *E. coli*'s outer membrane. The scientists hypothesized that increasing the level of CD14 in the milk would enhance protection.

"When inserted into the mammary gland through the opening of a cow's teats, CD14 binds to the *E. coli* and triggers the cow's immune response, which fights mastitis inflammation," says Hammond. "That process helps to neutralise and clear toxins produced by the bacteria, lessening the chances of an excessive immune response."

The researchers infused the CD14 protein into one of a test cow's four teats, or "quarters." All four quarters were subsequently exposed to *E. coli*. Fewer viable bacteria were recovered from the quarter that received the CD14 treatment than from those that did not receive the plant-derived protein.

A Top-Notch Protein Factory

The researchers chose tobacco plants, *Nicotiana benthamiana*, to be their CD14-producing factories. "We inoculated the young plants with laboratory-produced RNA of our recombinant virus by rubbing a small drop of the RNA onto the plants' leaves."

Once the viral RNA enters the test plants through small tears in the leaves, it begins to spread and the CD14 gene begins to make the protein. The protein can then be extracted from mashed-up leaves.

Hammond says this is the first report of a functionally active animal receptor protein being produced in a plant.

When a plant is infected with a virus, thousands of copies of viral RNA are made in each plant cell. "When our recombinant virus reproduces itself in a plant cell, it also makes the target protein, CD14. This is how the virus turns a plant into a bio-factory that rapidly generates proteins of interest," says Nemchinov. Separating and extracting the therapeutic protein from the host plant is possible because Nemchinov first tagged the CD14 protein with the amino acid histidine. "The histamine-tag tracker enables us to harvest high levels of the desired plant-produced protein," he says.

The researchers are able to purify about 1,000 micrograms of CD14 from 10 grams of leaf tissue taken from one plant. That means each of these plants provides enough protein to potentially treat about 10 cows with a dosage of 100 micrograms each. Fifty plants would yield purified protein to treat a herd of 500 cows.

One large greenhouse can accommodate enough host plants for large-scale purification of therapeutic protein. Another advantage of the greenhouse approach is that the plants inoculated with laboratory-derived infectious RNA could be used to inoculate more plants to scale-up protein production.

Partnering for Further Development

ARS has applied for patent protection on the plant-derived CD14, and the researchers are now seeking partners to help further develop and test the protein for safety, effectiveness, and proper dosage.

The CD14-based product may eventually be commercially developed for use by dairy farmers as a treatment to prevent cows from becoming infected during their dry period. Dairy cows are milked for 305 days and then enter a 60-day dry period, during which they are most susceptible to coliform infections. The plant-made CD14 could be incorporated into a polymer and infused into the udder during dry-off. The polymer would allow slow release throughout the dry period to help fight infections.

"As a next step, we'd like to work with a commercial partner to produce large volumes of plant-made CD14 and then conduct further tests to determine the most effective dosages in cows to achieve maximal protection from infection," says Hammond. "We may not need as much as the 100 micrograms per dose that we used in our first tests. Further studies may show that we can achieve the same results with less protein."

By expressing an easily purified therapeutic protein in plants, the ARS team has developed a novel preventive approach to treating mastitis that may provide a cost-effective alternative to antibiotic use.

Hyperspectral Imaging: A Non-Invasive Technique

Consumers have shown a willingness to pay a premium for guaranteed tender steaks. To increase consumer satisfaction and value of beef, the industry has a strong interest in tenderness predictors. An accurate, noninvasive, online tenderness instrument is needed for packing plant scenarios. Since beef carcasses are quality and yield graded by USDA employees two days postmortem, and product typically reaches the consumer at 14 days postmortem, the machine would need to accurately predict the ultimate 14 day postmortem tenderness value.

Hyperspectral imaging is a technique whereby multiple reflectance images are captured at regular intervals along a spectral axis. Thus, each pixel in a hyperspectral image has spectral reflectance data. In contrast, near-infrared (NIR) spectroscopy measures spectral reflectance of an entire field of view rather than a single pixel. Thus, hyperspectral imaging would be expected to be much more accurate as a result of the additional information that is captured.

The objective of this research project was to develop and validate an accurate, noninvasive tenderness predictor by scanning steaks at 14 days postmortem to then ultimately develop a system to predict the 14 day tenderness level (tender, intermediate, or tough) by scanning steaks at two day postmortem.

Procedure

Hyperspectral Imaging Apparatus

A hyperspectral imaging apparatus was constructed by integrating a CCD digital video camera (Model: IPX- 2M30, Imperx Inc., Boca

Raton, FL) and a spectrograph (Model: Enhanced series Imspector, Specim, Finland). The spectrograph has a spectral range of 400-1,000 nm. Spatial and spectral calibrations were performed. A diffuse-flood lighting system was designed using tungsten-halogen lamps and a dome with a white reflectance coating. Lighting was provided with six 50-W tungsten halogen lamps (Model: MR16, Phillips Lighting Co.). A lamp controller (Model: TXC300-72/120, Mercron Industries, Richardson, Tex.) converted 60 Hz AC voltage to 60 kHz. At this high frequency, tungsten halogen lamps do not respond quickly. This simulates a constant DC voltage power supply. Over the lifespan, tungsten halogen lamps get dimmer. A photodiode was placed near a tungsten halogen lamp that provides feedback to the controller. Based on the feedback, the current input to tungsten halogen lamps is increased to provide a constant intensity output. Over the lamps, a hemispherical dome of 40 cm diametre was placed, providing uniform diffuse light over the steak.

USDA Choice and Select grade longissimus steaks from between the 12th and 13th ribs and cut to 1-inch thickness were placed on metal trays which were then vacuum packaged. The trays contained 6-14 steaks and were placed in a commercial refrigerator for a 24 hour thawing time to an internal temperature of 1-6°C. Steaks and a white reference plate were then placed on a Teflon-coated plate mounted on a linear slide that used a stepper motor for movement.

The steak was then scanned by the camera to obtain a three-dimensional data cube (reflectance by two dimensional position). Scanning takes approximately 30 seconds to collect the image, and each file is approximately 600 mb. Images were obtained at wavelength intervals of 2 nm. Steaks were then cooked immediately on an impingement oven to an internal temperature of 69.5-72.2°C, and slice shear force values were obtained within one minute by an Instron Texture Analyser.

Statistical Analysis

A 200 by 300 pixel region of the image was selected for analysis. The region of interest was in the approximate location where slice shear force samples were obtained. Principal component analysis was carried out to reduce the dimension along the spectral axis. Over 90% of the variance of all bands in the image was explained by the first five principal components. The first four principle components are shown. On each principal component image, co-occurrence matrix analysis was conducted to extract eight image-textural features; thus a total of 40 image-textural features were actually obtained from each steak. To reduce the number of features and predict 3 tenderness categories (tender - slice shear force 21 kg; intermediate 21.1 to 25.9 kg; tough 26 kg), a canonical discriminant model was developed. Leave-oneout cross validation procedures were implemented to predict the tenderness level.

Results

The model correctly classified 9 tender, nine intermediate, and five tough samples, incorrectly classified three intermediate samples as tender, and incorrectly classified one tender sample as intermediate. All tough samples were correctly identified. Tenderness was predicted by this hyperspectral imaging device with 96.4% accuracy (Table 1).

Implications

This hyperspectral imaging system was effective in accurately predicting 14 day tenderness of beef longissimus steaks. With implementation of a non-invasive, accurate tenderness predictor, beef cuts could be labelled and sold at a premium as guaranteed tender. With this premium, producers, feedlots and packing plants would reap the benefits together.

Pelvic Measurements and Calving Difficulty

Calving Difficulty

Calving difficulty results in major economic loss to the beef cattle industry. Estimated losses resulting from dystocia (calving difficulty) equal or exceed $750,000,000 annually. Calving difficulty influences the economics of a cow/calf enterprise through increased calf death loss, increased labour and veterinary costs, reduced subsequent reproductive performance of the cow, potential loss of the cow, and reduced milk production.

Calf mortality may be four to eight times greater in dystocia cases than in normal births. The majority of calf deaths occur within the first 24 hours following calving (58 percent), with 75 percent of the total occurring within the first week of life. Studies indicate that calf death loss due to dystocia accounts for the single largest perinatal and postnatal death loss category through the first 96 hours after birth. A number of factors affect calving difficulty, including:

- Birth weight of the calf
- Pelvic area of the cow

- Gestation length
- Sex of calf
- Inadequacies in heifer development
- Body condition of the cow at calving
- Abnormalities in hormone profiles at the time of birth
- Abnormal presentation of the calf at birth.

We also know that the single major cause of dystocia is a disproportion between size of the calf at birth (birth weight) and the cow's birth canal (pelvic area). Differences in pelvic area are generally due to pelvic height, with discrepancies between the dam and fetus more likely to occur for pelvic height and depth of calf chest than for width measures.

Pelvic size, independent of cow weight, affects calving difficulty. Heifers of increased skeletal size usually have larger pelvic openings, but also tend to have heavier calves at birth. Hence, selection for cow size alone is ineffective.

Heifer weight and age generally have a positive relationship to pelvic area, but weight is not always a good indicator. External dimensions such as width of hooks and length of rump are not good indicators of pelvic area or calving difficulty. For these reasons pelvic measurements can be a useful management tool to eliminate heifers with a higher potential for calving difficulty.

Pelvic Measurements

University of Nebraska researchers developed ratios that you may use to estimate deliverable calf size. You can divide total pelvic area prior to breeding by a ratio that is based on age and weight to estimate the amount of birth weight a heifer could accommodate as a 2-year-old without substantial difficulty.

Example: A 600-pound yearling heifer (Table 1) with a pelvic area of 140 sq cm should be able to deliver, as a 2-year-old, a 67-pound calf without difficulty ($140/2.1 = 67$).

Pelvic measurements can be obtained at the time of pregnancy exam, but a factor of 2.7 should be used to estimate calf birth weight of 18- to 19-month-old 800-pound heifers. Tables 1 and 2 provide estimates of the deliverable calf size a heifer can accommodate at first calving based on pelvic area at given weights and ages. Scientists at the University of Nebraska suggest that these ratios appear to be good indicators of dystocia and report an accuracy of nearly 80 percent.

Structural traits in cattle tend to be highly heritable and pelvic area is no exception. This means there is a large genetic influence on pelvic area, which results in rapid response to selection. However, pelvic area is genetically correlated with many other traits, so selection for increased pelvic area alone can result in other traits changing for the worse. For example, selecting for increased pelvic area can result in increased birth weight and mature weight.

Pelvic measurements can be taken prior to the first breeding season and combined with a reproductive tract examination. Pelvic measurements should be used in addition to, not in place of, selection for size, weight, and above all, fertility. Producers should be aware that selection for pelvic area is likely to result in increased size of the entire skeleton and animal. Increased skeletal size of the dam will be reflected in higher birth weight and dimensions of the calf.

Pelvic measurements, on the other hand, can be used to successfully identify abnormally small or abnormally shaped pelvises. These situations, if left unidentified, are often associated with extreme dystocia, resulting in Cesarean delivery and even death of the calf or cow.

Pelvic measurements can be obtained with a Rice Pelvimetre, manufactured by Lane Manufacturing, 2075 South Valencia, Unit C, Denver, CO 80231; the Krautmann-Litton Bovine Pelvic Metre, manufactured Jorgensen Labs, Inc., 2198 West 15th St., Loveland, CO 80538; or the Equibov Bovine Pelvimetre, manufactured by Equibov, 205 Harris Street, Rockwood, Ontario, CAN NOB2KO.

The vertical measurement is the vertical diametre between the symphysis pubis on the floor of the pelvis and the sacral vertebrae. The horizontal measurement is obtained by determining the horizontal diametre at its widest point between the left and right ileal shafts. These measurements are read in centimetres and multiplied together to obtain the total pelvic area in square centimetres.

Measurements may be obtained by a veterinarian or an experienced producer. It is important that the person doing the measuring have a thorough understanding of the birth canal, pelvic structure, and reproductive tract. Practice and experience are necessary before accurate measurements can be obtained.

Summary

Calving ease will continue to be an important consideration as the industry produces fast-growing muscular progeny by terminal sires. These sires should be selected on measures of direct calving ease by using EPD (expected progeny difference) values for calving ease and birth weight.

To accommodate fairly heavy birth weights, scientists at Colorado State University recommend that you develop a cow herd that excels in maternal calving ease. Sires of replacement females should be selected to maintain cow size and milk production at levels compatible with available resources.

In addition, cows should be selected for total maternal calving ease along with gestation length.

Research indicates that bigger is not necessarily better when one considers actual pelvic measurements. In other words, heifers with large pelvic measurements fail to calve more easily than average-sized heifers. However, heifers with abnormally small pelvises or abnormally shaped pelvises generally experience a higher than normal incidence of calving difficulty and should be identified and culled from the herd.

Remember, pelvic area and shape are only a part of the calving difficulty complex. Follow the suggestions in the following list to minimise the incidence and severity of calving difficulty in your herd. How to reduce calving difficulty (in ranked order):

1. Breed heifers to proven calving ease bulls (low birth-weight EPDs)

2. Develop heifers to prebreeding target weights.

3. Ensure that heifers are in good body condition going into the calving period (minimum body condition score of 5).

4. Obtain pelvic measurements at yearling age and cull heifers with abnormally shaped or abnormally small pelvic areas.

A Blueprint for Eradicating Bovine TB

Over the course of the year 2008, bovine tuberculosis infected over 500 new herds in the UK and led to the slaughter of over four and a half thousand cattle. Despite of continuous prevention strategies, this figure presents a sharp increase from the year before. The economic cost of the disease has also soared in recent years, from £7.3 million in the year 1998/9 to £32.6 million in 2007/08.

Struggling to get to grips with the ever-worsening effects of the disease, the TB Advisory Group published a final report on the possibility of complete eradication within the UK.

Released April 8 2009, the report - Bovine Tuberculosis in England: Towards Eradication - April 2009 - is a conclusion of almost three years work in which the Group says it played a key role in obtaining stakeholder buy-in to TB control policies, independently challenged Government and considered issues of concern to stakeholders whilst advising on practical implementation of control policies.

In the Direction of a Wind of Change

The UK recently saw the proposed legislation of a badger cull fail on the grounds of animal welfare. This has left many in the role of TB control feeling deflated and at a loss for ideas of where to turn next.

The report emphasises the need to reinstate a sense of urgency, ensuring sufficient resources are available for this to become possible. It also makes it clear that there is 'no magic bullet' for eventual control and eradication. All attempts must be made to minimise the disease transmission risk and a consistent risk reduction approach must be used for all breakdowns.

According to the report, a "holistic multifaceted approach" is needed that uses a combination of control measures. For the TB Advisory Group's plan of action to succeed they say that substantial extra costs must be incurred and a realistic time frame between 10 and 20 years must be allowed for any hope of complete eradication.

The plan must also take into account TB existing in wildlife reservoirs. The report says that the plan will need to "stop the spread of Bovine TB from existing endemic areas", and also "Stamp out the disease where it occurs in new areas."

Another area that the reports highlights is to dispel the myths and misconceptions that many farmers have over the nature of the disease. "Who communicates this message is paramount and veterinary endorsement is key", says the report. Similarly the importance of this goal can not be lost due to set backs and promises of an easier future. A badger vaccine will not provide an instant cure, says the report. It will be used merely as part of the multifaceted approach.

Most importantly, clear leadership from both the government and the industry needs to materialise.

Chapter 2

Examining Key Issues and Details

The body of the Advisory Groups proposal was laid out in a set of key issues, which were aimed at controlling the current TB situation. Due to the rapid potential spread of the disease, control of cattle movement was of high importance, but as the industry relies on a considerable amount of trade to function, the report also emphasised that careful consideration must be used to evaluate the extent of these measures.

Current movement schemes follow control measures designed to prevent the spread of Foot and Mouth Disease, but the advisory group deemed these to be ineffective against Bovine TB. According to the report, a new specific set of measures must be implemented to help properly safeguard herds against infection.

Testing programmes were another key issue that fell under the group's scrutiny. They were "not convinced" of the clarity on the government's TB policy, whether it aimed to control, or eradicate the disease. According to the report, the initial objective must be to control the disease. Clearer objectives have been recommended with possible targets to underpin levels of progress.

The advisory group also discussed the conflicting opinions on pre-movement and post-movement testing. The group says that it supported the pre-movement testing policy as a means of reducing the risk of TB spread, but felt that more time was needed to see the epidemiological impacts of the measure. However, the group also acknowledged that a greater risk of wider disease spread is associated with cattle movements. Therefore the group decided that post-movement testing was more relevant for animals moving on to farms with breeding herds because of the "potentially greater consequences of introduction of infection into such herds."

As part of its recommendations on testing the group suggested that Defra should amend its current policy to fully comply with a council directive which states that all standard inconclusive reactors to the skin test must be slaughtered.

The directive also says that Member States may employ the gamma interferon blood test alongside the skin test to enhance the sensitivity of the diagnostic regime. The advisory group welcomed this suggestion and said that the test should be made more widely available, despite of extra costs plus legal and logistical issues.

Despite of the imposed and upheld ban on badger culls, the report still identifies the importance of badger populations to the plan. In the absence of culling, the report recommends tightened biosecurity measures, whilst future vaccination will play a key role in disease control and even possible eradication. It is currently believed that a licensed injectable badger vaccine will become available in 2010, so it is important that those involved in the issue start to develop a plan for successful deployment. The report also notes the importance of other possible wildlife reservoirs and advises continued research into these areas.

Husbandry was another issue that the group felt vital for good biosecurity. The tailoring of advice to specific TB outbreaks was deemed to be of great importance, whilst education on basic control measures and even the associated terminology was recommended. For instance the report believed there was widespread misunderstanding of the word biosecurity, as a result the group have advocated the use of the phrase "disease risk reduction measures" in place of it.

The report identified many misunderstandings about Bovine TB and recommended that veterinarians should make a greater effort to inform livestock keepers of the situation. "Whilst this would improve future communications there is a need to address current shortfalls in knowledge and general; misunderstandings, and some changes in terminology could be beneficial" .

As part of these measures the group stressed the importance of ensuring that feed stores, cattle housing and feeding areas are made out of bounds to wildlife - especially badgers - as far as practicable. Having isolation units was also considered to be good practice.

On the implementation of current controls the report acknowledged the current review of the testing process and welcomed the tightening of audit process and the increased control. The group has also heard from farmers and veterinarians of the dangers in undertaking TB testing and accepted the requirement for proper handling facilities for safety.

Controlling Mastitis in the Herd

According to Dr Andrew Bradley from Quality Milk Management Services Ltd the overall incidence of mastitis are also decreasing together with the somatic cell counts in herds.

In a study of 1,845 herds taken over three years for the prevalence of sub-clinical mastitis, it was found that for 45 per cent of the herd the somatic cell count was above 200,000 cells per ml.

In 25 per cent of the herds, more than 30 per cent of the cow readings were above 200,000 cells per ml and more than 20 per cent of the cows remained above 200,000 cells per ml for two consecutive recordings.

However, he said that studies show that there is a movement away from the cause of sub-clinical mastitis being from Staphylococcus aureus - contagious mastitis transmitted from cow to cow - and an increase in the cause being Streptococcus uberis - an environmental cause.

When studies looked at the prevalence of clinical mastitis, it was found that while there had been programmes in the UK for 20 years to control the problem, now things had started to slip back.

However, he said that the studies had found that there is no relationship between the herd size and bulk-milk somatic-cell count (BMSCC). The shift, he said was from contagious to environmental pathogens.

He said that planned programmes have done a lot to improve mastitis on farms and also improve milk quality and the main principles of mastitis control were to remove the existing infections and prevent new ones.

"As long as the rate of cure and culling exceeds the rate of new infection then progress will be made," he said.

However, he added that do not only have to remove existing infections but they need to address the underlying problems and the source of potential new infections.

One major question that has to be addressed is whether it is better to control the mastitis during lactation or during the dry period.

In looking at the prevalence during the dry period, it was found that there were large amounts during the first and second months of lactation.

He said that the controls for mastitis are very different for the dry period and for the period during lactation and understanding this aspect and getting to correct controls was a crucial part of understanding mastitis and prioritising controls on the farm.

An effective on farm plan needs to address all aspects of mastitis control and it needs to focus on prevention and not cure, Dr Bradley said.

The controls also need to be farm specific and there also needs to be an on-going commitment from the farmer to incorporate ongoing monitor=ring outcomes.

In the UK, he advised the farmers to adopt control plans, such as those organised and administered by the industry body Dairy Co.

DR Bradley added that it is also essential to take the appropriate choices in treatment to be effective. Rapid identification is crucial and the critical time is at the first milking. If it is missed once, the cure rate drops by 50 per cent, he said.

The aim must be to achieve a bacteriological cure although a cure can be affected by the strain of the pathogen and if the pathogen is resistant to penicillin or has an antibiotic resistance.

The effectiveness also depends on the ICSCC (cell count), the number of quarters affected in the animal and the udder pathology and well as the timing of infection - whether it is during the dry period or during lactation and the type and duration of the treatment.

For the herd, the cell count and the prevalence of different pathogens as well as the likelihood of new infections will also affect treatment.

The major requirement for control of mastitis are to understand what mastitis control means and the farmer needs to work closely with the vet and advisors to ensure an effective plan is put in place.

Although treatment plays a part, it is not the key and control measures are also important and successful controls rely on monitoring the outcomes of control measures.

Understanding the Ruminant Animal's Digestive System

Ruminant livestock include cattle, sheep and goats. Ruminants are hoofed mammals that have a unique digestive system that allows them to better use energy from fibrous plant material than other herbivores.

Unlike monogastrics such as swine and poultry, ruminants have a digestive system designed to ferment feedstuffs and provide precursors for energy for the animal to use. By better understanding how the digestive system of the ruminant works, livestock producers can better understand how to care for and feed ruminant animals.

Ruminant Digestive Anatomy and Function

The ruminant digestive system uniquely qualifies ruminant animals such as cattle to efficiently use high roughage feedstuffs, including forages. Anatomy of the ruminant digestive system includes the mouth, tongue, salivary glands (producing saliva for buffering rumen pH), esophagus, four compartment stomach (rumen, reticulum, omasum, and abomasum), pancreas, gall bladder, small intestine (duodenum, jejunum, and ileum), and large intestine (cecum, colon, and rectum).

A ruminant uses its mouth (oral cavity) and tongue to harvest forages during grazing or to consume harvested feedstuffs. Cattle harvest forages during grazing by wrapping their tongues around the plants and then pulling to tear the forage for consumption. On average, cattle take from 25,000 to more than 40,000 prehensile bites to harvest forage while grazing each day. They typically spend more than one-third of their time grazing, one-third of their time ruminating (cud chewing), and slightly less than one-third of their time idling where they are, neither grazing nor ruminating.

The roof of the ruminant mouth is a hard/soft palate without incisors. The lower jaw incisors work against this hard dental pad. The incisors of grass/roughage selectors are wide with a shovel-shaped crown, while those of concentrate selectors are narrower and chiselshaped. Premolars and molars match between upper and lower jaws. These teeth crush and grind plant material during initial chewing and rumination.

Saliva aids in chewing and swallowing, contains enzymes for breakdown of fat (salivary lipase) and starch (salivary amylase), and is involved in nitrogen recycling to the rumen. Saliva's most important function is to buffer pH levels in the reticulum and rumen. A mature cow produces up to 50 quarts of saliva per day, but this varies, depending on the amount of time spent chewing feed, because that stimulates saliva production.

Forage and feed mixes with saliva containing sodium, potassium, phosphate, bicarbonate, and urea when consumed, to form a bolus. That bolus then moves from the mouth to the reticulum through a tube-like passage called the esophagus. Muscle contractions and pressure differences carry these substances down the esophagus to the reticulum.

Ruminants eat rapidly, swallowing much of their feedstuffs without chewing it sufficiently (< 1.5 inches). The esophagus functions bidirectionally in ruminants, allowing them to regurgitate their cud for further chewing, if necessary. The process of rumination or "chewing the cud" is where forage and other feedstuffs are forced back to the mouth for further chewing and mixing with saliva.

This cud is then swallowed again and passed into the reticulum. Then the solid portion slowly moves into the rumen for fermentation, while most of the liquid portion rapidly moves from the reticulorumen into the omasum and then abomasum. The solid portion left behind in the rumen typically remains for up to 48 hours and forms a dense mat in the rumen, where microbes can use the fibrous feedstuffs to make precursors for energy.

True ruminants, such as cattle, sheep, goats, deer, and antelope, have one stomach with four compartments: the rumen, reticulum, omasum, and abomasums. The ruminant stomach occupies almost 75 percent of the abdominal cavity, filling nearly all of the left side and extending significantly into the right side. The relative size of the four compartments is as follows: the rumen and reticulum comprise 84 percent of the volume of the total stomach, the omasum 12 percent, and the abomasum 4 percent. The rumen is the largest stomach compartment, holding up to 40 gallons in a mature cow.

The reticulum holds approximately 5 gallons in the mature cow. Typically, the rumen and reticulum are considered one organ because they have similar functions and are separated only by a small muscular fold of tissue. They are collectively referred to as the reticulorumen. The omasum and abomasum hold up to 15 and 7 gallons, respectively, in the mature cow.

The reticulorumen is home to a population of microorganisms (microbes or "rumen bugs") that include bacteria, protozoa, and fungi. These microbes ferment and break down plant cell walls into their carbohydrate fractions and produce volatile fatty acids (VFAs), such as acetate (used for fat synthesis), priopionate (used for glucose synthesis), and butyrate from these carbohydrates. The animal later uses these VFAs for energy.

The reticulum is called the "honeycomb" because of the honeycomb appearance of its lining. It sits underneath and toward the front of the rumen, lying against the diaphragm. Ingesta flow freely between the reticulum and rumen. The main function of the reticulum is to collect smaller digesta particles and move them into the omasum, while the larger particles remain in the rumen for further digestion.

The reticulum also traps and collects heavy/dense objects the animal consumes. When a ruminant consumes a nail, wire, or other sharp heavy object, it is very likely the object will be caught in the reticulum. During normal digestive tract contractions, this object can penetrate the reticulum wall and make its way to the heart, where it can lead to hardware disease. The reticulum is sometimes referred to as the "hardware stomach." Hardware disease is discussed in detail in Mississippi State University Extension Service Publication 2519, "Beef Cattle Nutritional Disorders."

The rumen is sometimes called the "paunch." It is lined with papillae for nutrient absorption and divided by muscular pillars into the dorsal, ventral, caudodorsal, and caudoventral sacs. The rumen acts as a fermentation vat by hosting microbial fermentation. About 50 to 65 percent of starch and soluble sugar consumed is digested in the rumen. Rumen microorganisms (primarily bacteria) digest cellulose from plant cell walls, digest complex starch, synthesize protein from nonprotein nitrogen, and synthesize B vitamins and vitamin K. Rumen pH typically ranges from 6.5 to 6.8. The rumen environment is anaerobic (without oxygen). Gases produced in the rumen include carbon dioxide, methane, and hydrogen sulfide. The gas fraction rises to the top of the rumen above the liquid fraction.

The omasum is spherical and connected to the reticulum by a short tunnel. It is called the "many piles" or the "butcher's bible" in reference to the many folds or leaves that resemble pages of a book. These folds increase the surface area, which increases the area that absorbs nutrients from feed and water. Water absorption occurs in the omasum. Cattle have a highly developed, large omasum.

The abomasum is the "true stomach" of a ruminant. It is the compartment that is most similar to a stomach in a nonruminant. The abomasum produces hydrochloric acid and digestive enzymes, such as pepsin (breaks down proteins), and receives digestive enzymes secreted from the pancreas, such as pancreatic lipase (breaks down fats). These secretions help prepare proteins for absorption in the intestines. The pH in the abomasum generally ranges from 3.5 to 4.0. The chief cells in the abomasum secrete mucous to protect the abomasal wall from acid damage.

The small and large intestines follow the abomasum as further sites of nutrient absorption. The small intestine is a tube up to 150 feet long with a 20-gallon capacity in a mature cow. Digesta entering the small intestine mix with secretions from the pancreas and liver, which elevate the pH from 2.5 to between 7 and 8. This higher pH is needed for enzymes in the small intestine to work properly. Bile from the gall bladder is secreted into the first section of the small intestine, the duodenum, to aid in digestion. Active nutrient absorption occurs throughout the small intestine, including rumen bypass protein absorption.

The intestinal wall contains numerous "finger-like" projections called villi that increase intestinal surface area to aid in nutrient absorption. Muscular contractions aid in mixing digesta and moving it to the next section.

The large intestine absorbs water from material passing through it and then excretes the remaining material as feces from the rectum. The cecum is a large blind pouch at the beginning of the large intestine, approximately 3 feet long with a 2-gallon capacity in the mature cow. The cecum serves little function in a ruminant, unlike its role in horses. The colon is the site of most of the water absorption in the large intestine.

Ruminant Digestive Development

Immature ruminants, such as young, growing calves from birth to about 2 to 3 months of age, are functionally nonruminants. The reticular groove (sometimes referred to as esophageal groove) in these young animals is formed by muscular folds of the reticulum. It shunts milk directly to the omasum and then abomasum, bypassing the reticulorumen. The rumen in these animals must be inoculated with rumen microorganisms, including bacteria, fungi, and protozoa. This is thought to be accomplished through mature ruminants licking calves and environmental contact with these microorganisms.

Immature ruminants must undergo reticulorumenomasal growth, including increases in volume and muscle. In a calf at birth, the abomasum is the largest compartment of the stomach, making up more than 50 percent of the total stomach area. The reticulorumen and omasum account for 35 percent and 14 percent of the total stomach area in the newborn calf. As ruminants develop, the reticulorumen and omasum grow rapidly and account for increasing proportions of the total stomach area. In mature cattle, the abomasum encompasses only 21 percent of the total stomach capacity, whereas the reticulorumen and omasum make up 62 and 24 percent, respectively, of the total stomach area. Rumen papillae (sites of nutrient absorption) lengthen and decrease in numbers as part of rumen development.

Because immature ruminants do not have a functional rumen, feeding recommendations differ for developing ruminants compared with adult ruminants. For instance, it is recommended immature ruminants are not allowed access to feeds containing non-protein nitrogen such as urea. Developing ruminants are also more sensitive to gossypol and dietary fat levels than mature ruminants. Design nutritional programs for ruminants considering animal age.

Ruminant Feeding Types

Based on the diets they prefer, ruminants can be classified into distinct feeding types: concentrate selectors, grass/roughage eaters, and intermediate types. The relative sizes of various digestive system organs differ by ruminant feeding type, creating differences in feeding adaptations. Knowledge of grazing preferences and adaptations amongst ruminant livestock species helps in planning grazing systems for each individual species and also for multiple species grazed together or on the same acreage.

Concentrate selectors have a small reticulorumen in relation to body size and selectively browse trees and shrubs. Deer and giraffes are examples of concentrate selectors. Animals in this group of ruminants select plants and plant parts high in easily digestible, nutrient dense substances such as plant starch, protein, and fat. For example, deer prefer legumes over grasses. Concentrate selectors are very limited in their ability to digest the fibres and cellulose in plant cell walls. Grass/roughage eaters (bulk and roughage eaters) include cattle and sheep. These ruminants depend on diets of grasses and other fibrous plant material. They prefer diets of fresh grasses over legumes but can adequately manage rapidly fermenting feedstuffs. Grass/roughage eaters have much longer intestines relative to body length and a shorter proportion of large intestine to small intestine as compared with concentrate selectors.

Goats are classified as intermediate types and prefer forbs and browse such as woody, shrubby type plants. This group of ruminants has adaptations of both concentrate selectors and grass/roughage eaters. They have a fair though limited capacity to digest cellulose in plant cell walls.

Carbohydrate Digestion

Forages

On high-forage diets ruminants often ruminate or regurgitate ingested forage. This allows them to "chew their cud" to reduce particle size and improve digestibility. As ruminants are transitioned to higher concentrate (grain-based) diets, they ruminate less.

Once inside the reticulorumen, forage is exposed to a unique population of microbes that begin to ferment and digest the plant cell wall components and break these components down into carbohydrates and sugars. Rumen microbes use carbohydrates along with ammonia and amino acids to grow. The microbes ferment sugars to produce VFAs (acetate, propionate, butyrate), methane, hydrogen sulfide, and carbon dioxide. The VFAs are then absorbed across the rumen wall, where they go to the liver. Once at the liver, the VFAs are converted to glucose via gluconeogenesis. Because plant cell walls are slow to digest, this acid production is very slow. Coupled with routine rumination (chewing and rechewing of the cud) that increases salivary flow, this makes for a rather stable pH environment (around 6.0).

Hight - Concentrate Feedstuffs (Grain)

When ruminants are fed high-grain or concentrate rations, the digestion process is similar to forage digestion, with a few exceptions. Typically, on a high-grain diet, there is less chewing and ruminating, which leads to less salivary production and buffering agents' being produced. Additionally, most grains have a high concentration of readily digestible carbohydrates, unlike the more structural carbohydrates found in plant cell walls. This readily digestible carbohydrate is rapidly digested, resulting in an increase in VFA production. The relative concentrations of the VFAs are also changed, with propionate being produced in the greatest quantity, followed by acetate and butyrate. Less methane and heat are produced as well. The increase in VFA production leads to a more acidic environment (pH 5.5). It also causes a shift in the microbial population by decreasing the forage using microbial population and potentially leading to a decrease in digestibility of forages.

Lactic acid, a strong acid, is a byproduct of starch fermentation. Lactic acid production, coupled with the increased VFA production, can overwhelm the ruminant's ability to buffer and absorb those acids and lead to metabolic acidosis. The acidic environment leads to tissue damage within the rumen and can lead to ulcerations of the rumen wall. Take care to provide adequate forage and avoid situations that might lead to acidosis when feeding ruminants high-concentrate diets. Acidosis is discussed in detail in Mississippi State University Extension Service Publication 2519, "Beef Cattle Nutritional Disorders." In addition, energy as a nutrient in ruminant diets is discussed in detail in Mississippi State University Extension Service Publication 2504, "Energy in Beef Cattle Diets."

Protein Digestion

Two sources of protein are available for the ruminant to use: protein from feed and microbial protein from the microbes that inhabit its rumen. A ruminant is unique in that it has a symbiotic relationship with these microbes.

Like other living creatures, these microbes have requirements for protein and energy to facilitate growth and reproduction. During digestive contractions, some of these microorganisms are "washed" out of the rumen into the abomasum where they are digested like other proteins, thereby creating a source of protein for the animal.

All crude protein (CP) the animal ingests is divided into two fractions, degradable intake protein (DIP) and undegradable intake protein (UIP, also called "rumen bypass protein"). Each feedstuff (such as cottonseed meal, soybean hulls, and annual ryegrass forage) has different proportions of each protein type. Rumen microbes break down the DIP into ammonia (NH_3) amino acids, and peptides, which are used by the microbes along with energy from carbohydrate digestion for growth and reproduction.

Excess ammonia is absorbed via the rumen wall and converted into urea in the liver, where it returns in the blood to the saliva or is excreted by the body. Urea toxicity comes from overfeeding urea to ruminants. Ingested urea is immediately degraded to ammonia in the rumen.

When more ammonia than energy is available for building protein from the nitrogen supplied by urea, the excess ammonia is absorbed through the rumen wall. Toxicity occurs when the excess ammonia overwhelms the liver's ability to detoxify it into urea. This can kill the animal. However, with sufficient energy, microbes use ammonia and amino acids to grow and reproduce.

The rumen does not degrade the UIP component of feedstuffs. The UIP "bypasses" the rumen and makes its way from the omasum to the abomasum. In the abomasum, the ruminant uses UIP along with microorganisms washed out of the rumen as a protein source. Protein as a nutrient in ruminant diets is discussed in detail in Mississippi State University Extension Service Publication 2499, "Protein in Beef Cattle Diets."

Importance of Ruminant Livestock

Importance of Ruminant Livestock The digestive system of ruminants optimizes use of rumen microbe fermentation products. This adaptation lets ruminants use resources (such as high-fibre forage) that cannot be used by or are not available to other animals. Ruminants are in a unique position of being able to use such resources that are not in demand by humans but in turn provide man with a vital food source. Ruminants are also useful in converting vast renewable resources from pasture into other products for human use such as hides, fertilizer, and other inedible products (such as horns and bone).

One of the best ways to improve agricultural sustainability is by developing and using effective ruminant livestock grazing systems. More than 60 percent of the land area in the world is too poor or erodible for cultivation but can become productive when used for ruminant grazing. Ruminant livestock can use land for grazing that would otherwise not be suitable for crop production. Ruminant livestock production also complements crop production, because ruminants can use the byproducts of these crop systems that are not in demand for human use or consumption. Developing a good understanding of ruminant digestive anatomy and function can help livestock producers better plan appropriate nutritional programs and properly manage ruminant animals in various production systems.

Controlling BVDV - First Steps

It causes significant gastrointestinal, respiratory and reproductive disease in cattle Dr Dan Givens from the Auburn University College of Veterinary Medicine told the recent US National Cattlemen's Beef Association Convention.

He said that if an infection reaches 34 per cent of a herd, losses have been estimated at $20 per calving if it is a low virulent strain and this can go up to $57 per calving if the strain is highly virulent.

The losses could be even higher because of hidden loss, such as suppression of the immune system, or low fertility caused by BVDV.

He said the significance of the disease could be seen by the large number of different vaccines that are on the market - estimated at more than 180. However, Dr Givens said that vaccination is only half the answer, as vaccinating cows can only cannot completely protect developing foetuses from infection and the calves can act as reservoirs for BVDV and remain carriers for the rest of their life.

If foetuses are infected with BVDV in the first 150 days of gestation, then they risk being aborted or their immune system can be altered so that they have the viral infection for life.

Dr Givens said that these infected animals shed a lot of infectious viruses through faeces, urine, saliva, nasal discharge, hair and secretions from the reproductive tract. These animals which hold a persistent infection are more common than many people believe, Dr Givens said, and they are a critical link in the continued transmission of viruses and they are a continual economic burden on the business.

He showed that numerous tests on herds in the US and in the UK among beef and dairy herds had shown a prevalence of persistently infected animals ranging from under one per cent (3 out of 1,769 tested in the UK) to more than 10 per cent (59 out of 559 tested in Wyoming in the US).

Identification and Removal

Apart from vaccination, these persistently infected animals need to be removed, to control BVDV, and to do this the herds need to be tested regularly to identify the infected animals.

The producer can work out a strategy for controlling BVDV by working out a testing programme together with the vets.

DR Givens said that there are also ELISA (enzyme linked immunoabsorbent assay) tests that can be carried out on ear notches after the sample has either been frozen or refrigerated. There are also immunohistochemistry tests that can be carried out on samples in formalin. Dr Givens said that thee tests are not affected by ingestion of maternal antibodies in colostrums, so they can be carried out on animals under six months old. An antigen capture serum test, which isolates the virus from serum, can be affected by the ingestion of maternal antibodies, so it should be carried out on calves over six months old. However, Dr Givens added that while the tests are reliable, no test is perfect and if a positive reaction is found then the animals should be retested in 21 days to verify whether the calf is BVDV positive or not.

VLA Reports Oncrease in Calf Problems

Weather and Climate

Late November and December were extremely cold and there were sub-zero temperatures and widespread snow-cover across much of GB for several weeks. One consequence of this was the need to feed livestock additional forage and as a result forage supplies on many farms became rapidly depleted. This could have an adverse effect on cattle nutrition this winter, and will also increase the cost of production.

Scanning Surveillance Submission Numbers

In England and Wales in the fourth quarter of 2010 there was a decrease in the total number of diagnostic submissions and of carcases in particular, compared to Q4 of 2008 and 2009; although there was little observed difference in submissions for 2010 as a whole. The decrease in submissions for Q4 was probably due to three factors:

- Increase in charges to private veterinary surgeons, particularly for necropsies.

- Introduction of a triage procedure to avoid necropsy on submissions where diagnosis could be made by testing of samples.

- Extensive snow in December.

Compared to Q4 of 2009, the reduction in submissions occurred in all regions of GB and in both beef and dairy cattle.

For the year, the number of submissions examined for scanning surveillance was similar to that in 2009. Slightly fewer carcases were necropsied in E&W (for the reasons above) but more were done in Scotland.

Figure 1

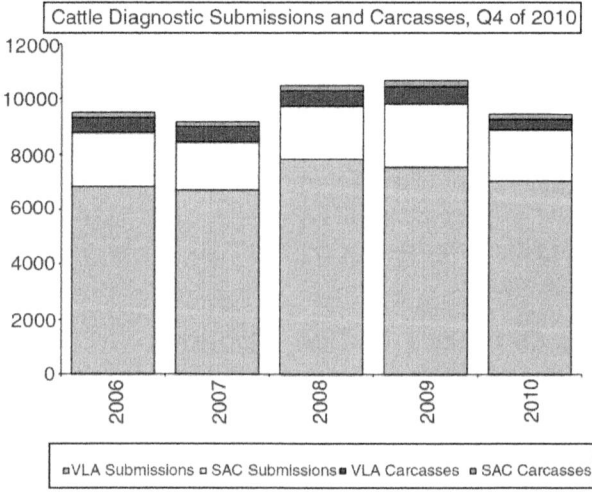

Figure 1.

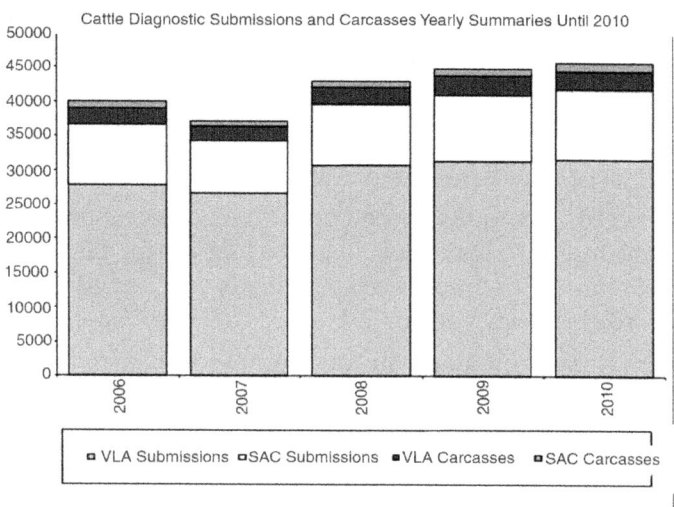

Figure 2.

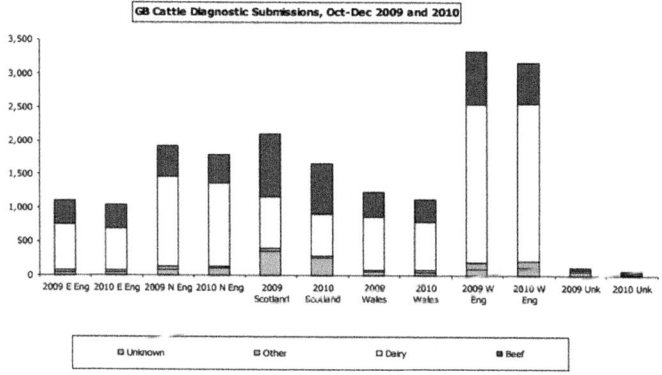

Figure 3.

New and Emerging Diseases Identified in the Quarter

Analysis of Diagnosis Not Reached (DNR)

During 2010, 25per cent of cattle submissions in GB were undiagnosed; similar to previous years (26per cent). However, at 23per cent, the per centDNR for the final quarter of 2010 (October – December) was significantly lower than Q4 in previous years (26per cent) and Q3 in 2010 (27per cent).

Conversely, a statistically significant increase in undiagnosed skin cases occurred during Q4 2010. However, given the small number of incidents (n=10) and that these incidents were of many different clinical presentations of skin disease, there was no suggestion of an undiagnosed, emerging skin condition. Monitoring will continue and no further action is warranted.

The increase in undiagnosed enteric disease reported in Q3 2010 did not continue into Q4 and the annual figure for 2010 indicated an overall decrease in undiagnosed enteric disease across the age groups compared to previous years.

Similarly the increase in undiagnosed respiratory disease in English and Welsh cattle observed in September 2010 did not continue into the final quarter of the year. Monitoring will continue with no further action advised at this stage.

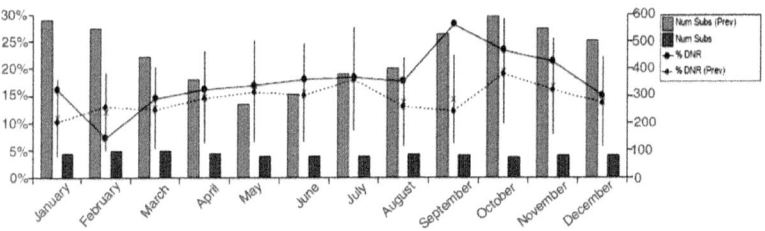

Figure 4: Comparison of cases of undiagnosed cases respiratory disease in England and Wales in 2010 with previous years.

On-going New and Emerging Disease Investigations

Metritis in a Dairy Herd

This project was undertaken in a 400 cow dairy herd with a rising incidence of metritis cases manifested by a purulent vaginal discharge in the first three weeks after calving. The purpose of the project was to investigate the potential role of bacteria and viruses (Bovine Herpes Virus-4, BoHV-4 and Bovine Lymphocytic Herpes Virus, BLHV). Fifteen clinically affected and fifteen unaffected animals were selected and sampled by the private veterinary surgeon. Metritis was strongly associated with the isolation of *Arcanobacterium pyogenes* from vaginal swabs, as previously reported, and *Histophilus somni* and *Streptococcus pluranimalium* were isolated from vaginal swabs from both groups of animals.

BLHV was detected in similar numbers of affected and unaffected animals. Whilst detection of BoHV-4 in blood was equally common in both groups, the virus was only detected in vaginal swabs from animals in the clinically affected group. An opportunistic or synergistic role for this agent could not be ruled out. The preliminary findings were presented at the BCVA Congress in October (Welchman and others (2010) Cattle Practice 18 (2), 136-137). Currently, the results indicate an association (not necessarily causal) between metritis and the presence of *A. pyogenes* and also of BoHV-4 in vaginal discharges. However, analysis of the results is underway to determine the significance of these associations.

Bibersteinia Trehalosi in Cattle

The increased frequency of isolation of the bacterium *Bibersteinia trehalosi* from cattle was first reported in our Second Quarter, 2009 report, and again in the Third Quarter, 2010 report. As this is a recognised commensal and pathogen of sheep, we wish to determine if the isolates associated with disease in cattle are likely to have common from sheep or are cattle-specific. Both ovine and bovine isolates have been submitted, together with geographical data, Glasgow University for molecular typing. Results are awaited.

Acute Holstein Haemorrhage Syndrome

This syndrome will be discussed at the European Pathology Discussion Group meeting at Lasswade on March 16th 2011. There will be a joint presentation by Tim Crawshaw (VLA Starcross), Mark Wessels (VLA Preston) and Cathy Lamb (Glasgow University). The investigation protocol will be given to the assembled European pathologists with a view to fostering international collaboration on the investigation.

Chapter 3

Unusual Diagnoses

Negated Cases of Suspected Abortion due to Brucellosis

Modified acid fast organisms were identified in bovine placental material on two occasions during this quarter. On one occasion, bacilli smaller than Brucella or Coxiella burnetii were identified as the bacterium *Psychrobacter phenylpyruvicus*. This organism is ubiquitous in the environment but can cause opportunistic human infection. It is a gram-negative organism with cell-wall surface lipopolysaccharides that share cross-reactive epitopes with *Brucella sp*. Although there was a placentitis it wasn't clear whether this organism had caused the disease leading to the abortion. On another occasion acid fast organisms were seen intracellularly from a placental smear but PCR ruled out *Chlamydophila* and *Coxiella burnetii*.

Both of these are rare occurrences with little impact for state veterinary medicine. It does emphasise the efficiency of the scanning surveillance activities of the VLA in ruling out the possibility of *Coxiella burnetii* – a zoonotic infection, and *Brucella abortus* which is a notifiable disease.

Changes in Disease Patterns and Risk Factors

Annual Trend: Salmonellosis

A statistically significant annual increase in salmonellosis of serotypes excluding S. Typhimurium and S Dublin was observed in 2010. This involved England and Wales, but not Scotland.

In the first and third quarters, S Mbandaka was identified as the predominant serotype, affecting mainly adult dairy cattle in the southwest of England. This serotype is associated with feeding 'straights' such as soya and rapeseed meal. The reason for the increase is unclear and would require further study to elucidate. The risk is two-fold: disease in cattle and disease in humans.

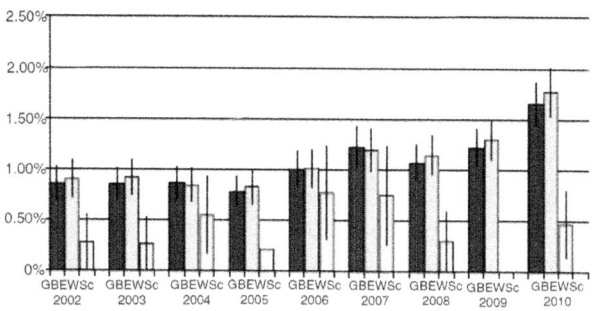

Figure 1: Annual diagnoses of salmonellosis (excluding S Typhimurium and S Dublin) in GB, E&W & Scotland

For cattle, the impact in terms of morbidity and mortality, for these salmonelloses is low. Currently, the number of incidents in cattle is also relatively low. There were 230 scanning surveillance diagnoses of salmonellosis caused by serotypes other than other than S. Typhimurium and S. Dublin in 2010. This is an increase from 99 incidents in 2005. However, a very small proportion of GB cattle are affected. The risk to public health from salmonella in cattle is believed to be low, because of low prevalence in cattle and measures to prevent contamination of the food chain.

The trend will be monitored through 2011 and, should it continue, will be investigated in order to determine the specific risk factors associated with S. Mbandaka.

Fasciolosis

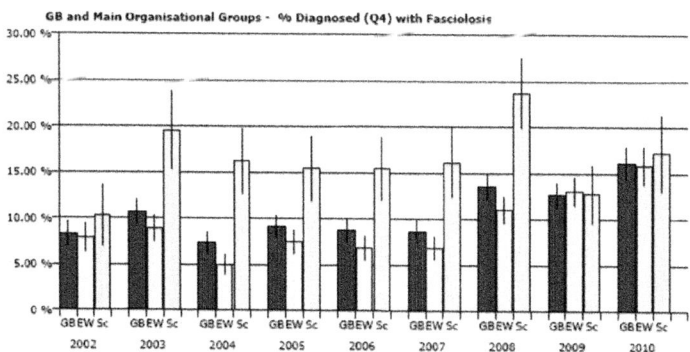

Figure 2: Annual diagnoses of fasciolosis in GB, E&W & Scotland

There was a significant rise in the percentage diagnosis of fasciolosis in GB for the fourth quarter compared to the same quarter in 2009.

The reason for this rise is not immediately apparent. There was a moderate forecast for fasciolosis for 2010 based on lower rainfall last spring and summer, which was 84per cent of the thirty-year average between 1971 and 2000 for England and Wales, and 69per cent for Scotland.

Farmers may have been less inclined to incur the cost of treatment, based on the 20, there was a forecast for significant disease.

The trend will continue to be monitored, but promotion of herd health plans, such as the VLA's Herdsure for liver fluke, is the best, long term-means of controlling fasciolosis in dairy and beef herds.

Neonatal Calf Diarrhoea

Diarrhoea is a common disease in young beef and dairy calves. It is a cause of considerable economic loss, impairs welfare significantly and results in widespread use of, sometimes undesirable, antibiotic therapy.

Rotavirus infection and cryptosporidiosis are the two major infectious causes and both increased in England and Wales in 2010.

The proportion of diagnoses of rotavirus infection, although significantly greater in this quarter than the fourth quarter of 2009, is not dissimilar from that of previous years.

This is not the case for cryptosporidiosis, for which there were significantly more diagnoses in 2010 than in any of the preceding recent years. The cryptosporidiosis trend has been reported to industry levy-funded bodies in GB.

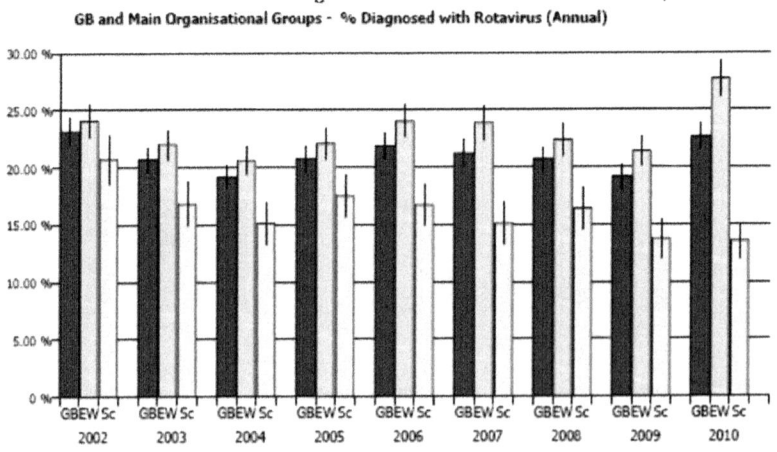

Figure 3: Annual diagnoses of rotavirus infection in GB, E&W & Scotland

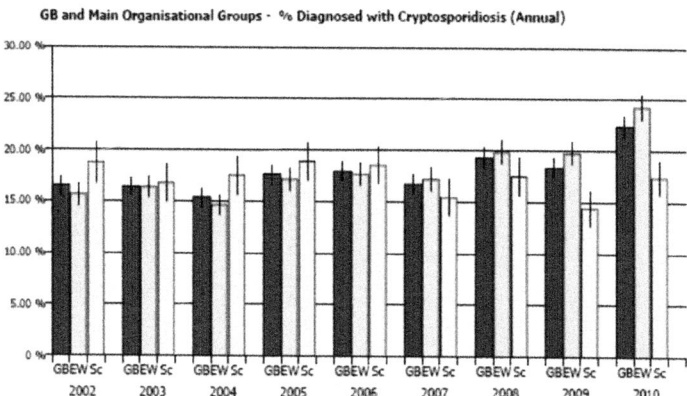

GB and Main Organisational Groups - % Diagnosed with Cryptosporidiosis (Annual)

Figure 4: Annual diagnoses of cryptosporidiosis in GB, E&W & Scotland

The actual numbers of diagnoses increased, as well as the proportion of samples tested yielding a diagnosis: cryptosporidiosis – 2009=1,278' 2010=1,562; rotavirus - 2009=1,059, 2010=1,214.

The factors responsible for the observed increase in diagnoses of cryptosporidiosis are not fully understood. Cryptosporidiosis is spread by the faeco-oral route, with persistence in the environment. Therefore factors associated with faecal hygiene of calf housing and pastures are likely to be involved. It could be beneficial to know whether failure to control cryptosporidiosis was due to lack of awareness of existing control measures, awareness but lack of implementation, or implementation but lack of efficacy. This could be an area for further research and has been suggested to industry bodies.

The VLA is currently undertaking some work on cryptosporidiosis:

- Farm-level studies on a small number of farms, with the intention of identifying the risk factors associated with the disease;

- Further work on the association between animal and human disease, to determine how much of the latter originates in animals.

Johne's Disease

As of the 1st of October 2010, serology has replaced microscopy as the primary diagnostic test for Johne's disease. As serology has greater sensitivity, this could influence trends in scanning surveillance data on JD and changes from this date require appropriate interpretation. However, there was no significant change in the proportion of diagnostic submissions yielding a diagnosis of Johne's disease for Q4 2010.

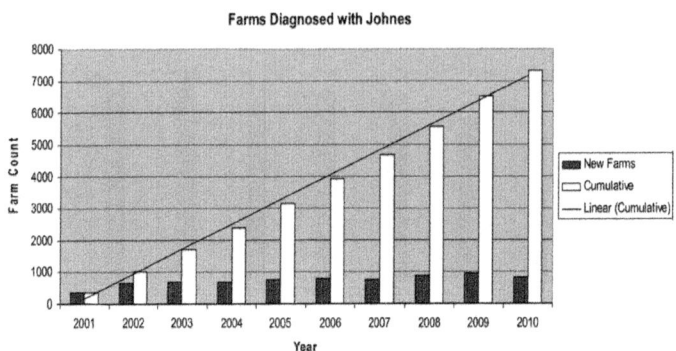

Figure 5: Number of farms in GB in which Johne's disease was diagnosed

Horizon-scanning

Economics of the Beef Cattle Industry

The June census for 2010 indicated a slight rise of 2.8per cent in the numbers of adult females in the national beef herd for England. In Wales there was a 2per cent rise in the number of non-dairy breeding female animals from 237,000 to 242,000. This small increase in breeding females suggests that there will be a continued supply of beef cattle to market for 2011. The greatest threat to the beef industry in 2011 will be the rising price of commodities, such as concentrate and grain feed and fuel costs, which will probably continue during 2011. This will reduce the profit margin of beef farmers. Farmers may seek to make economies by reducing the involvement of their veterinary practices, which could adversely affect scanning surveillance.

Economics of the Dairy Cattle Industry

Although the milk price has remained relatively stable, the price of several farm inputs has risen sharply: feed wheat costs nearly twice as much as 12 months ago, oil seed rape prices are very high and there is a shortage of reasonably priced good quality forage and straw.

It is likely that we see more effects of the above later in the winter of 2010/11, in particular if turn out is delayed. The higher input prices may adversely affect cash flow on dairy farms and hence may have a negative effect on the number of submissions. This effect may be partly off-set by an on-going shortage of dairy heifers: high stock prices encourage the investigation of disease.

Beef Cattle Breeding

A number of pharmaceutical companies are investing in genomics of cattle (including the genetic analysis of animal susceptibility to disease) to assess future breeding potential and suitability for artificial insemination. Genomic analysis provides information of these traits much sooner compared to, for example, assessing progeny performance for beef bulls used for artificial insemination. Genomic analysis for disease susceptibility is at an advanced stage for feedlot-reared cattle in the United States. There is also growing interest from -beef producers in this country and evaluation of beef cattle genomics may have a significant effect on the health of beef cattle in GB. The first case of in the UK was diagnosed in April, since then 77 calves on 51 farms across England and Wales have been diagnosed with the disease. Cases of the disease have also been reported in Germany, Belgium and the Netherlands, since 2008. The disease is also known in France and Italy. The Netherlands has reported more than a hundred dead calves due to the disease.

Bleeding Calf Syndrome: The Facts

The first case of in the UK was diagnosed in April, since then 77 calves on 51 farms across England and Wales have been diagnosed with the disease. Cases of the disease have also been reported in Germany, Belgium and the Netherlands, since 2008. The disease is also known in France and Italy. The Netherlands has reported more than a hundred dead calves due to the disease.

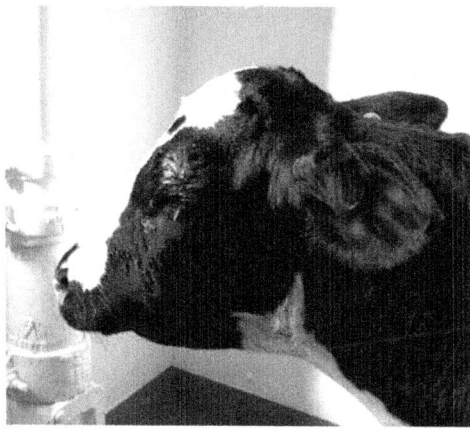

Figure 6: Bleeding from the head

What does the Disease Look Like?

Clinical signs in calves include bleeding from apparently intact skin and also from injection and ear tagging sites together with signs of bleeding from visible mucous membranes, nose and rectum. There may be intestinal bleeding, with calves passing dark, tarry dung. Calves are also noticed to have a high fever.

What Causes the Disease?

The symptoms are caused by an almost complete destruction of the bone marrow of the calf which produces the red and white blood cells vital for the animal's immune system and blood clotting mechanisms. This seems to be occurring at or around the time of birth, although it is uncertain whether the damage is occurring in the womb or soon after birth.

The cause is not yet known. There are a number of lines of investigation which are being pursued, which include management and environmental factors on the affected farms. Although there is currently no evidence of an infectious cause it cannot be totally ruled out at this point.

Does the Disease Lead to Death?

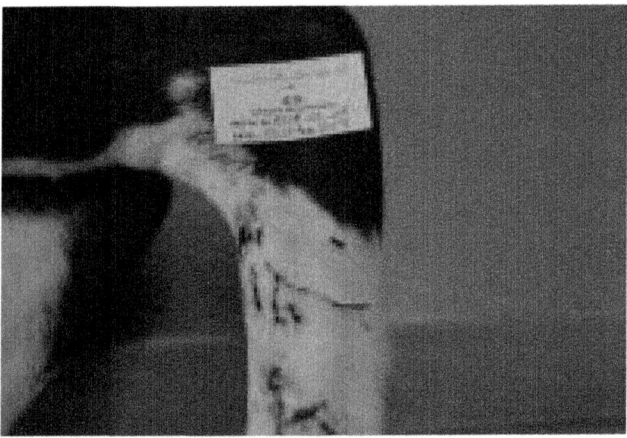

Figure 7: Bleeding from the hind limb

Only a few calves have been affected in any one herd, but once affected they usually die. The mortality rate of calves with the disease is about 95 per cent, there are reports, mainly anecdotal, of some affected calves making a full recovery.

Only calves less than four weeks old are affected. The mothers of the affected calves are usually perfectly healthy.

Is there Any Risk to Humans Through Contact or Food?

As the age of the animal affected is 0 – 4 weeks, they would not be entering the food chain. The age they are affected is very consistent and the disease has never been seen in older animals. To date no infectious agent (known or novel) likely to have caused the condition has been identified in any of the tissues of affected calves.

There has been no direct evidence or reports of any potential transmission to people in Germany where the disease has been present for at least 18 months.

There is currently no evidence to suggest that the disease is infectious or contagious.

The Human Animal Infections and Risk Surveillance (HAIRS) group, which routinely meets to assess any risks to human health from emerging diseases, has been briefed and are considering the available data.

What is being Done to Find out More about the Disease?

Research carried out by VLA and Scottish Agricultural College (SAC), funded by Defra and the Scottish Government, is ongoing and is designed to identify the potential factors which might be causing the disease.

An international meeting is taking place in December to consider what is known about the condition and to identify the best way forward in collaborative investigation.

What should Farmers do if they See the Symptoms in their Herd?

They should consult their own vet who can submit calves to their local VLA or SAC laboratory for a full examination. To encourage farmers to get in touch with the authorities, SAC and VLA are offering a free post mortem service to farmers who have suspected cases. Blood samples from suspected live clinical cases are carried out free of charge.

Understanding Animal Health

Livestock diseases cause enormous losses through death and decreased production, impacting directly on food security and local economies. Their occurrence also hinders trade through restrictions on the movement of livestock commodities, especially at the international level. The Office International des Epizooties (OIE) estimates that animal disease may result in losses of up to 20% of production (OIE 1993). The majority of the population in most developing countries are involved in smallholder agriculture. Often this group also represents one of the poorest sectors of society. In addition to food and draft power, livestock represent an important savings system within the village economy.

In such countries, diseases of livestock have serious effects at many levels, especially as they are usually more severe, more widespread, and inflict more social and economic damage than in developed countries. At the same time, the resources available to identify, assess and control these diseases are often scarce. For this reason, it is important that any resources available are effectively targeted to achieve the most benefit.

Accurate information about the health status of a nation's animal population is critical in the fight against animal diseases. Without measures of the frequency and economic importance of a particular disease, a government's task of targeting disease control is almost impossible. Without comprehensive disease reporting systems and ongoing measures of disease frequency, the efficacy and endpoint of any control or eradication program is impossible to measure. Without an internationally acceptable system of epidemiological surveillance and animal health information management, the verification of national freedom from disease or a disease-free zone is impossible to achieve.

Unfortunately, in many developing countries the systems in place for the collection, management and reporting of animal health information are not able to gather the type of information that is required for informed priority setting; disease control program planning, implementation and evaluation; and substantiation of claims of freedom from disease. This is despite sometimes substantial investment in veterinary infrastructure and disease control activities, such as laboratory diagnostic facilities and vaccination programs. Consequently, issues relevant to the design and development of animal health information systems are attracting attention in both developed and (in particular) in developing countries. This book is a contribution to this research area.

What is an Animal Health Information System?

There is a growing recognition among veterinary administrators throughout the world of the need for more quantitative and reliable information on livestock production and disease. Better information is critical to efficient and effective disease control as well as becoming increasingly important in certification for international trade in livestock and livestock products. Some countries have, and many are moving towards developing, national animal health information systems with data being derived from a number of sources.

The problem with many existing data sources is that, because of nonreporting and under-reporting, they are statistically biased and do not give a fair picture of the situation in the reference population (McCallon and Beal 1982; Hueston 1993). The need for additional, representative information obtained through active surveillance is now well recognised in both the human and veterinary fields. Indeed, it may be argued that in many developing countries, the information needs of animal health authorities can, for the foreseeable future, only be met by active surveillance. A national animal health information system is the complete system responsible for handling information about the health of livestock in a country. Such a system may include systems for some or all of the following purposes:

The Approach Taken in this Book

The overall goal of the research described in this book was to develop and evaluate the tools necessary to provide decision-makers with reliable animal health information placed in context and analysed appropriately. This goal was achieved by:

1. The collection of information including
   - disease reports,
   - livestock population data,
   - vaccine production, distribution and delivery,
   - livestock movements,
   - meat inspection findings, and
   - active surveillance for the collection of unbiased disease data;
2. Recording the information collected, preferably with a set of standard forms containing all the required information;
3. Transmitting that information to centres for compilation;
4. Managing that information efficiently (a computerised database);
5. Entering the data into the computer (data entry staff);
6. Analysing and mapping the data (statistical and mapping software);
7. Reporting the data (computerised report formats);
8. Communicating the results of analyses to decision-makers;

9. Using the reported data to take action on the basis of the information provided; and

10. Feedback of reported data converted to meaningful information to all levels of staff and contributors who provided it.

Thus, a national animal health information system is not merely a computerised database as is sometimes thought. Rather, it is the entire process of gathering, managing, analysing and reporting information in accordance with the needs of a particular country. Traditionally such a system has been based around what has been termed passive surveillance— essentially 'waiting' for existing and new diseases to be detected somewhere in the system. In many situations resource constraints (especially financial) may hinder attempts to improve the passive surveillance-based system as a whole. The research reported in this book argues that a more focused, active surveillance-based approach using information technology, where appropriate, can achieve significant across-the-board advances in the performance of animal health information systems in developing countries.

Improved Laboratory Procedures

While laboratory procedures were not a significant problem in Thailand (compared to many developing countries) there was still considerable room for improvement, especially if support for an active surveillance-based program was required. Thus, of improved laboratory techniques and quality control procedures developed for the diagnosis of hog cholera, Aujeszky's disease and infectious bursal disease, three new rapid antigen detection and three new serological tests for antibody detection were implemented at the Northern Veterinary Research and Diagnostic Centre (NVRDC) in Lampang, northern Thailand. These quality control procedures meet international ISO (International Standards Organisation) 9000 specifications and are now in routine use in the NVRDC virology laboratory.

The antigen detection tests have considerable advantages over former technology including improved convenience, reduced cost, improved accuracy, and a dramatic reduction in time to diagnosis (e.g. a reduction from 3–4 weeks to 3–8 hours in the case of Aujeszky's disease and hog cholera). This improvement in diagnostic ability means that diagnoses can now be provided in time to influence decisions on interventions rather than merely being an historical confirmation of a clinically suspect event. The new serological tests have similar advantages with the addition of a marked increase in capacity which is vital for animal health monitoring. A quality control process for laboratory assays has been put in place and is now in routine use in the virology laboratory at the NVRDC and has also been introduced to the other regional laboratories in Thailand. The system is called 'QCEL' and has the following features:

- provides the user with an independent assessment on unacceptable trends in eznyme-linked immunosorbent assay (ELISA) performance;
- provides individual operator performance data;
- requires no assumed knowledge of statistics;
- gives easy-to-interpret graphical summaries of quality control data;
- uses international standard methods (Shewart-CUSUM); and is
- inexpensive, and simple to implement and use.

Improved Surveillance

Active surveillance methods were developed and evaluated in Thailand and Lao PDR. In Thailand, research towards this objective involved the development and testing of methodologies aimed at the collection of three core measures of disease: seroprevalence; disease incidence; and freedom from disease.

The approaches used to develop these methodologies involved: A review of the literature with regard to techniques previously used for the collection of the three core disease information types; A systematic assessment of the information requirements of the veterinary services An assessment of the current information collection capabilities and restraints faced by the veterinary services; Theoretical development of approaches to improved data collection; In some cases, stochastic simulation modelling to test the validity of the techniques; Training of field staff and implementation of survey techniques to field test the methodologies; and Critical analysis of both the effectiveness of the methodology and the data collected.

Seroprevalence Surveys

Research initially concentrated on the development of techniques for foot and mouth disease (FMD) surveillance and serological monitoring of the official vaccination program. The new techniques are now in routine use in northern Thailand.

Features of the technique include the following:

- A flexible methodology for serosurveillance applicable to virtually any developing country situation. This is achieved through the use of a two stage sampling approach, in which the first-stage (selection of villages or herds) can be modified according to the sampling frame available (ranging from a good quality sampling frame with reliable livestock population data, through to no sampling frame at all).

- A new approach to first-stage random sampling using random geographic coordinate sampling which allows the selection of a true random sample (of villages or herds) in the absence of a sampling frame. The new technique achieves greater accuracy at a lower cost than previously used techniques. The use of a geographical information system (GIS) simplifies the sampling process as well as introduces significant benefits in planning the logistics involved in field work; further benefits accrue if remotely sensed data (satellite images or aerial photographs) are available.

  Compilation (and testing through simulation) of formulae for minimum sample size estimation, tailored to the variance structures of different livestock populations (resulting in significant cost savings for routine surveys run as part of a monitoring program).

- A practical approach to the random selection of individual animals at the village level, effectively removing errors due to selection bias.

These techniques were successfully field tested in northern Thailand and validated in the Lao PDR and have since been implemented in other developing countries such as the Philippines.

Disease Incidence Estimation

Prevalence data only provides some of the information relevant to animal disease control. Disease incidence is the other key measure of disease required to monitor control program progress, and for international reporting. Two approaches to the estimation of disease incidence were developed. Both are based on the use of village interviews to collect reliable retrospective disease outbreak data quickly and inexpensively. A number of methods developed in the area of participatory rural appraisal were modified and adopted to ensure the quality of data recalled by livestock owners is the best possible.

The first technique applies backwards recurrence time analysis—an analytical technique akin to survival analysis borrowed from sociology—to calculate measures of disease occurrence. The second technique uses capture–recapture techniques (developed in the field of ecology) to calculate incidence estimates based on two data sources (combining, for example, laboratory submissions or disease reports with survey results).

Freedom from Disease

In order to reap the full benefits at the completion of disease control and eradication programs, developing countries must be able to demonstrate their freedom from disease. All trading countries are now required to provide soundly based evidence for their disease status. To support this, a new formula and survey approach was developed. The new probability formula is free from previous restrictive assumptions of a perfect diagnostic test or infinite population.

The techniques developed from the research program have proven their value to developing countries through extensive field testing. A package, known as *RapiCAPS*, was developed to bring the benefits of the research program to the developing country veterinary services that most need them. The package, a combination of computer software and a methodology manual, incorporates all the complex statistical and data manipulation routines required to successfully conduct the disease surveys developed in the research program, freeing developing country veterinarians from the need for access to high-level statistical consultants. While this is a useful advance in its own right, it also contributes directly to making the active surveillance approach more feasible for adoption and implementation in Southeast Asia and in developing countries generally. (*RapiCAPS* has been renamed the 'Survey Toolbox').

Longitudinal Studies

While small-scale livestock enterprises in villages are still the norm in Thailand, there is now an emerging small commercial sector, particularly in pigs. A series of longitudinal studies of selected diseases in representative herds were undertaken to measure their biological impact and identify critical factors relevant to control. Four small commercial piggeries and five poultry farms were enrolled in these studies. Blood samples collected during these studies were used to further evaluate the new diagnostic assays introduced to the NVRDC as part of the project. Analyses of the serological data confirmed the hog cholera ELISA and Aujeszky's disease latex agglutination tests were working well. In addition, serology was used to evaluate vaccination programs which were found to be deficient in some instances and corrective actions were taken.

Geographical Information System (GIS) Issues

For the sampling-based active surveillance to be effective, it is necessary to have as complete an understanding of the reference population as possible. This is required for drawing the samples, for executing the surveys and for placing the results in the wider national (or regional) context. It is also important to appreciate that much of this information is spatial in nature, therefore techniques developed in allied disciplines such as geographical sciences can make significant contribution.

The techniques developed from the research program have proven their value to developing countries through extensive field testing. A package, known as *RapiCAPS*, was developed to bring the benefits of the research program to the developing country veterinary services that most need them. The package, a combination of computer software and a methodology manual, incorporates all the complex statistical and data manipulation routines required to successfully conduct the disease surveys developed in the research program, freeing developing country veterinarians from the need for access to high-level statistical consultants. While this is a useful advance in its own right, it also contributes directly to making the active surveillance approach more feasible for adoption and implementation in Southeast Asia and in developing countries generally. (*RapiCAPS* has been renamed the 'Survey Toolbox').

Longitudinal Studies

While small-scale livestock enterprises in villages are still the norm in Thailand, there is now an emerging small commercial sector, particularly in pigs. A series of longitudinal studies of selected diseases in representative herds were undertaken to measure their biological impact and identify critical factors relevant to control. Four small commercial piggeries and five poultry farms were enrolled in these studies. Blood samples collected during these studies were used to further evaluate the new diagnostic assays introduced to the NVRDC as part of the project. Analyses of the serological data confirmed the hog cholera ELISA and Aujeszky's disease latex agglutination tests were working well. In addition, serology was used to evaluate vaccination programs which were found to be deficient in some instances and corrective actions were taken.

Geographical Information System (GIS) Issues

For the sampling-based active surveillance to be effective, it is necessary to have as complete an understanding of the reference population as possible. This is required for drawing the samples, for executing the surveys and for placing the results in the wider national (or regional) context. It is also important to appreciate that much of this information is spatial in nature, therefore techniques developed in allied disciplines such as geographical sciences can make significant contribution.

This rationale provided the impetus for research into the role of GISs and animal health information systems. Research issues investigated included identifying:

- the role of GISs in animal health systems generally;
- the problems involved in GIS development in a developing country;
- the role of the GIS in active surveillance; and
- identifying the role of the GIS in disease mapping and visualisation.

A major research effort was directed towards the development of an integrated data management system within a GIS framework suitable for collection, analysis and reporting of data at the local, regional and national levels. Research on the GIS-based information system involved a preliminary assessment of the current information flows and information requirements of different sectors of the veterinary authorities. This was followed by investigations into both the geographical information and attribute (animal health related) information that was already available, and identifying data that needed to be specially generated. At the commencement of the project only a rudimentary computer-based system was in existence in the Thai Department of Livestock Development (DLD)—this system had no GIS capabilities.

A model system was developed at the NVRDC based on three provinces (Lampang, Lamphun and Chiang Mai) in northern Thailand. This model system provided the basis for the further development of information technology for animal health information management by the DLD. The GIS application was based on *pcARC/INFO* (later *ArcView*) as the central software packages—both are dominant packages worldwide. This computer system, when linked to the existing disease database at the NVRDC, provided the capability of producing computerised maps of disease distributions in the pilot area to assist with the evaluation of the need for such technology in the DLD. Once basic computerised mapping capabilities had been established at the NVRDC, more sophisticated spatial analysis techniques (e.g. animated maps modelling disease outbreaks over time) were utilised for the analysis of animal health data.

Development of the pilot GIS demonstrated that incorporation of this technology into the DLD's animal health information system was quite feasible. The focus of the GIS component of the project in the latter part of the project shifted to making the system more sustainable. More DLD staff were trained in the use of the GIS to give them the capacity, if required, to expand the coverage to other parts of Thailand. This expansion meant that both the NVRDC and the Southern Veterinary Research and Diagnostic Centre (SVRDC) would have fully operational GIS capabilities in addition to expertise and facilities within the epidemiology unit at the National Institute for Animal Health in Bangkok for integration of the system at a national level. The GIS studies have also shown that the accuracy of the existing laboratory accession database could be enhanced through use of predefined codes and some drop-down menu systems; they have also demonstrated the geographical bias in the origin of current laboratory data.

An additional focus of the GIS component of the project was the development of output formats of maps and reports (both on screen and in hardcopy) relevant to DLD needs. These included the production of different map formats for displaying the distribution of livestock diseases, spatio-temporal visualisation of disease occurrence, disease outbreak management, and use of the GIS for producing village random samples for active surveillance of livestock diseases of interest.

Economic Issues

The research undertaken included a cost–benefit study of the economic impacts of FMD and the costs and benefits of eradication, in terms of the various impact categories. The economic evaluation of the Thai FMD control and eradication program indicated a number of factors which will help to assure success of the program and be of assistance to Thai livestock authorities in disease control policy formulation.

Economic analysis frameworks were developed for animal health economics. Data were collected from village surveys, discussions with Thai livestock officers, Thai official statistics, and modelling approaches.

Costs of livestock diseases were examined at the producer level and aggregated to the national level, with the addition of wider socioeconomic variables for policy making. Multi-stage sampling designs for active surveillance of seroprevalence levels against foot-and-mouth disease were evaluated in terms of cost-effectiveness using a simulation approach.

Information about costs of FMD in Thailand, costs of vaccination and other control measures and potential benefits of FMD eradication were integrated in a cost–benefit evaluation of the current Thai control and eradication program. This analysis integrated findings of other components of the project, and developed and applied a methodology for estimation of the net present value and benefit-to-cost payoff of the current Thai FMD control and eradication program. The analysis provides indicative results that the program has a positive net present value and a benefit-to-cost ratio exceeding unity. Provided current control measures are continued and adapted as necessary, the Thai FMD program appears to be well justified when all categories of benefits (including reduced animal health expenditure, trade gains, transport, and draught and animal welfare benefits) are taken into account. The importance of FMD eradication in Thailand becomes greater when viewed within a program of eradication in Southeast Asia. The economics related research inquiries may be grouped as follows.

Theoretical Models of Animal Health Economics

Optimal disease control effort. The earlier analyses of McInerney and others based on a loss–expenditure tradeoff were considered to be inappropriate for infectious diseases where a threshold expenditure was needed to make progress in disease control. This implied that the optimal control expenditure on a disease may be zero or a very high level, rather than some intermediate point such as may be optimal with a disease such as mastitis. Economic analyses indicate that this reasoning would appear to apply to FMD control in Thailand.

Models of economic benefits (economic surplus) for disease control programs. Traditional economic models have been extended to take account not only of producer benefits, but impacts on traders, consumers of livestock products, government fiscal impacts, and trade gains from expanded foreign markets. The theoretical conditions for maximising economic gain (e.g. in terms of demand elasticities) were explored and identified. This conceptual analysis has been incorporated into a cost–benefit analysis of FMD control in Thailand.

Applied Models of Animal Health Economics

Data were collected from various sources to develop profiles of livestock (the meat cattle and buffalo, dairy, pig and poultry) industries in Thailand, as a background to investigating production benefits and trade opportunities from improved animal health.

These reports have examined livestock numbers, management systems and disease status. Unlike cattle and buffalo, the pig and poultry industries have clearly defined commercial and village sectors, and disease control in the latter presents considerable difficulty (e.g. the cyclical nature of village pig production raises difficulties for regular vaccination against FMD).

As an understanding of socioeconomic aspects is important in predicting the success of animal health intervention measures by government, it was necessary to carry out socioeconomic analyses of the role of livestock in villages using cross-sectional survey data. The roles of women and of common property resources in the management of Thai village livestock production systems were also examined. In macroeconomic analysis of livestock industries, a closed general equilibrium (CGE) model was applied to examine the relationship between output of the livestock sector (as influenced by disease control measures) and other Thai industries.

Economics of Animal Health Information Systems Development

This research focused on cost-effective multi-stage sampling designs for active surveillance of FMD protection status. The World Health Organisation recommended design of 30 villages and 7 subjects (in this case, animals) from each was found to be quite robust to variations in population protection status and sampling cost parameters. In active surveillance for FMD (tests of seroprevalence), there was a tendency for 'natural' optima to arise with respect to sampling designs, due to cost discontinuities.

Separate from the economic evaluation of the economic benefits of animal health programs was the issue of the economic evaluation of the prototype GIS system which has been developed for three northern provinces in Thailand. While this GIS work has demonstrated how to overcome various obstacles in development of a modern information system for animal health, the expenditure incurred by it would be different from that for a national 'production' system of animal health information. As key details of information system costs were not collected or available it was not possible to carry out this economic assessment.

Conclusion

A new strategy for animal health information system research in Southeast Asia is reported in this book. Information technology-based active surveillance (including GIS) forms the core of this strategy. The methodology was developed in northern Thailand and tested under relatively more difficult conditions in the Lao PDR.

Principles of Disease Investigation and Surveillance in Livestock Systems

This paper discusses some of the basic elements necessary to provide good animal health information: investigation of disease occurrence; monitoring and surveillance; international guidelines; and animal health information systems. By understanding the basic epidemiology which creates disease patterns, livestock disease control authorities can undertake effective surveillance and control programs. Investigation of individual disease outbreaks requires a systematic set of procedures to help identify causes and source of the outbreak with a view to control and prevention of possible future ones. Disease surveillance is the continuous investigation of a given population to detect the occurrence of disease for control purposes.

The data for surveillance programs may be generated by a number of methods which include clinical evaluations, laboratory reports, slaughter inspection data, screening tests, or owner reports. The codes of the Office International des Epizooties include guidelines on surveillance and risk analysis which form the basis of quarantine strategies and health certification used to prevent the international spread of disease through the movement of animal commodities. Animal health information systems provide the data required to facilitate trade under international agreements. A good animal health information system should provide a reliable picture of the disease situation in a specified animal population. It should have a clear purpose and incorporate planned methods of data acquisition, management analysis and interpretation.

It is sometimes not appreciated that, although there are many chance elements in the spread of diseases in populations, the resultant patterns are not distributed randomly. Rather, these patterns have characteristics which can be observed and analysed to give a great deal of insight into the underlying processes. By understanding the basic epidemiology of diseases which create these patterns, livestock disease control authorities can undertake effective surveillance and control programs. However, identifying the pattern and understanding the principal driving processes is usually very difficult. The problem is that records of disease occurrence are frequently very sparse and lack the level of detail required to be able to detect the underlying pattern.

For infectious diseases particularly this situation is frequently exacerbated by the sensitivity of the information leading to lack of disclosure because of potential financial implications through loss of trade. However, this should not prevent disease control authorities from taking a scientific approach to disease investigation and surveillance. This paper discusses some of the basic elements necessary to provide good animal health information: investigation of disease occurrence; monitoring and surveillance; international guidelines; and animal health information systems.

Investigating Disease Outbreaks

This section gives an epidemiological perspective to disease outbreak investigations. An outbreak has been defined as a short-term epidemic or a series of disease events clustered in time and space. The disease events are usually new cases of a disease occurring at a higher frequency than that normally expected. Throughout this section the terms epidemic and outbreak are used more or less interchangeably. An outbreak investigation is a systematic procedure to help identify causes and sources of epidemics with a view to control of an existing epidemic and prevention of possible future ones. In most situations, the primary objective of an epidemic or disease outbreak investigation is to identify ways of preventing the further transmission of the disease-causing agent. The epidemiological approach to outbreak investigations is based on the premise that cases of a disease are *not* distributed randomly but occur in patterns within the at-risk population. It is the role of the epidemiologist to record and analyse these patterns to help meet the primary objective.

Nine Basic Steps

The procedure for an outbreak investigation follows nine basic steps. Not all steps are necessarily included in every investigation, nor do they always follow the same sequence. In practice, several steps will be undertaken simultaneously. The nine basic steps are: Each of these basic steps is further explained in the following sections.

The nine basic steps are:

1. Establish or verify the diagnosis.
2. Define a 'case'.

3. Confirm that an outbreak is actually occurring.

4. Characterise the outbreak in terms of time, animal and place. This step involves measuring disease frequency and documenting the patterns.

5. Analyse the data. This step involves calculating factor-specific attack rates and constructing an attack-rate table.

6. Formulate working hypotheses in an attempt to identify the type of epidemic, the possible source and mode of spread.

7. Undertake intensive follow-up investigations to identify high risk groups and possible further outbreaks.

8. Implement control and preventive measures.

9. Report the findings of the investigation with recommendations for dealing with future possible outbreaks of the same disease.

The Diagnosis

The initial provisional diagnosis in an outbreak is usually made on clinical signs, crude epidemiological patterns and gross pathology. Whenever possible, laboratory tests should be undertaken to verify the interim diagnosis. Since some laboratory procedures may require weeks to complete, the implementation of control measures is often based on the provisional diagnosis.

Define a Case

Where large numbers of animals are dying rapidly, such as with haemorrhagic septicaemia in a village or botulism in a large feedlot, a case will simply be a dead animal. The need to distinguish between the small number of deaths due to other causes is trivial in such situations. However, for many outbreaks specific criteria must be developed to define a case. These may be based on clinical, autopsy or laboratory findings. For example, in the bovine spongiform encephalopathy (BSE or 'mad cow disease') epidemic in the United Kingdom both clinical and histologically confirmed cases were used in studying the epidemic (Wilesmith et al. 1988).

A case may be based on part of an animal (e.g. the eye, limb or udder quarter), an individual animal or some aggregation of individuals such as a litter or herd. For example, with botulism in a feedlot a case is based on the individual affected animal but with Newcastle disease in smallholder chickens or foot-and-mouth disease a case may be an affected village. Where the disease aetiology is initially obscure it is better to have a fairly broad case definition to ensure that all likely cases are investigated. The case definition can be refined as more information comes to light and the data reanalysed accordingly.

Confirm the Outbreak

This step may seem superfluous but in many instances it is required, particularly where the disease is already endemic. For example, in many pig herds a certain level of pneumonia is expected but an undetected increase will lead to severe production deficits if not recognised early. By definition, an outbreak or epidemic exists when the current incidence is in excess of the usual incidence of cases in the population determined to be at risk. The term 'excess' is obviously imprecise. This is usually not an issue for large, common source epidemics but can pose a problem for either propagated or vector-borne diseases.

Time, Animal and Place

From an epidemiological viewpoint it is important to characterise the outbreak in terms of the above three variables for diseases where the cause is obscure. The characterisation must be done in such a manner that hypotheses can be developed regarding the source, mode of transmission and duration of the outbreak. The information is organised in an attempt to find answers to the following kinds of questions.

Time:

1. What is the exact period of the outbreak?
2. Given the diagnosis, what is the probable period of exposure?
3. Is the outbreak most likely common source, propagated or both?

Animal:

1. Are there any characteristics about groups of animals for which specific attack rates vary?
2. Which groups have the highest and which have the lowest attack rates?

Place:

1. What are the significant features of the geographical distribution of cases?
2. What are the relevant attack rates?

Time: Variation with time in the frequency of occurrence of cases of a disease is called its temporal pattern. There are three basic time spans used to describe disease temporal patterns: the epidemic period, which is of variable length depending on the duration of the particular epidemic; a 12 month period to describe seasonal patterns; and an indefinitely long period of years to identify long-term trends. A knowledge of seasonal patterns and long-term trends is important when deciding whether or not an epidemic exists in the present period and in predicting future epidemics. For example, foot-and mouth disease in some parts of Asia exhibits epidemic behaviour with a period of time, known as the inter-epidemic period, between epidemics. This is similar to many directly transmitted diseases which are highly contagious and produce a strong immunity in surviving animals.

The temporal pattern of an outbreak is described in terms of its epidemic curve. The epidemic curve is a graph showing the onset of cases of the disease in question either as a bar graph or frequency polygon. The first case identified for a particular outbreak is referred to as the *index* case. For infectious diseases, information about the index case can be valuable in ascertaining the source of the outbreak.

In general, an epidemic curve has four and sometimes five segments:

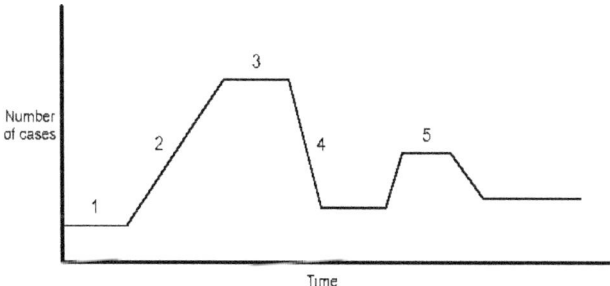

Figure 8. The five segments of a typical epidemic curve. (1) The endemic level; (2) an ascending branch; (3) a peak or plateau; (4) a descending branch; and (5) a secondary peak.

The slope of the ascending branch can indicate the type of exposure (propagating or common source) or the mode of transmission and incubation period of the disease agent. If transmission is rapid and the incubation period short, then the ascending branch will be steeper than if transmission is slow or if the incubation period is long. The length of the plateau and slope of the descending branch are related to the availability of susceptible animals which in turn is dependent on many factors such as stocking densities, the changing importance of different mechanisms of transmission and the proportion of immunes in the population at risk.

Secondary peaks are usually due to the introduction of new susceptibles or a change in the mode of transmission. For example, with botulism, toxico-infectious transmission may result in a long plateau, a descending branch with a gradual slope and secondary peaks in the outbreak. The interval of time chosen for graphing the cases is important to the subsequent interpretation of the epidemic curve. The time interval should be selected on the basis of the incubation or latency period of the disease and the period over which the cases are distributed. The appropriate time interval may vary from several hours (e.g. some acute intoxications) to a month or more (e.g. BSE).

A common error in this regard is the selection of a time interval that is too long. Overly long intervals obscure subtle differences in temporal patterns including secondary peaks resulting from animal to animal transmission. A rule of thumb is to make the interval between one eighth and one quarter as long as the incubation period. It may be wise to make several epidemic curves based on different graphing intervals and then select the one which best portrays the data. However, it should be remembered that in many disease outbreaks in animals the time of onset of illness is often obscure and compromises must be made when making epidemic curves.

The duration of an epidemic is influenced by:

- the number of susceptible animals exposed to a source of infection who become infected;
- the period of time over which susceptible animals are exposed to the source; and
- the minimum and maximum incubation periods of the disease.

Outbreaks involving a large number of cases—with opportunity for exposure limited to a day or less—of a disease having a maximum incubation period of a few days or less, usually have an epidemic curve which approximates a 'normal' distribution (symmetrical bell-shaped curve). Such epidemic curves usually indicate a common source origin with exposure over a short period relative to the maximum incubation period of the disease.

Animal

Although the word 'animal' is used here, we should really refer to cases and non-cases and their characteristics to embrace the wider definitions where cases might be herds etc. For simplicity, the discussion is restricted to animals only. Age, sex, geographical origin and genotype are frequently associated with varying risk of disease. However, it should be kept in mind that animal patterns can be closely linked to temporal and spatial patterns of disease. To describe patterns of disease by animal types, it is first necessary to outline what measures of disease frequency are used in outbreak investigations. The basic measure of disease frequency in outbreaks is the *attack rate* (AR). An attack rate is a special form of an incidence rate where the period of observation is relatively short.

An attack rate is the number of cases of the disease divided by the number of animals at risk at the beginning of the outbreak. Where different risk factors for the disease under investigation are to be evaluated, attack rates specific for the particular factor must be calculated. For example, say there were deaths of poultry in a village due to suspected hypervirulent infectious bursal disease (IBD) and it appeared that young birds were at greater risk of having IBD than adult birds. We might make the following calculations:

$$\text{For young birds, AR1} = \frac{\text{No. with IBD}}{\text{Total young birds}} \tag{1}$$

$$\text{For adult birds, AR2} = \frac{\text{No. with IBD}}{\text{Total adult birds}} \tag{2}$$

If some hypothetical numbers are used—say there were 1 000 young birds in the village and 300 died from IBD and there were 1 000 adult birds of which 100 died from IBD during the outbreak—the attack rates here are 30% and 10%, respectively, suggesting that young birds were three times more likely to die from IBD than adult birds. This finding could lend support to a hypothesis that young birds are more susceptible to infection, either because of their age or maybe because of their behaviour or maybe they have lower levels of immunity etc.

Formal measures to compare attack rates among groups of animals with different characteristics are described in the next section. With IBD of course the total number of birds in different risk categories would have to be estimated through representative sampling. Another problem could be the estimation of number dying and when they died.

Place

Describing the outbreak in terms of place may lead to the cause. For cattle in feedlots, this may involve looking at the pattern among different pens whereas in more extensive cattle operations, studying different paddocks or villages may yield important clues. It is often useful to consider place and time together. This can be done by drawing a plan of the pen, farm or village layout and recording the dates where cases occurred. Such a diagram may also give a lead to whether the outbreak is a common source or propagating. For larger scale epidemics, spot maps are useful.

Analysing the Data

Factor-specific attack rates for such factors as age, breed, sex, feed, pen, management system etc. are computed and arranged in an *attack rate table*. The higher the attack rate difference and the relative risk, the more important the specific factor is in increasing the risk of disease. The analysis becomes more complicated when trying to sort out the interactions and confounding among factors. Stratified and multivariate analyses are used to investigate these phenomena.

It should also be noted in the above example that chicks were three times more likely to have IBD than growers and six times more likely than adults. Also, growers were at twice the risk of adult birds. This dose–response phenomenon when relating size to attack rate lends support to the hypothesis that level of pre-existing immunity as manifested by age is a component 'cause' of IBD in this outbreak.

Working Hypotheses

Based on the analysis of time, place and animal data, working hypotheses are developed for further investigation. These may concern one or more of the following:

- whether the outbreak is common source or propagating;
- if a common source, whether it is a point or multiple exposure; and
- the mode of transmission—contact, vehicle or vector.

Any hypothesis should be compatible with all the facts. Corrective action can be taken based on the more realistic hypotheses. For example, the epidemiological analysis of the BSE epidemic in Great Britain (Wilesmith et al. 1988) suggested a common source epidemic consistent with the hypothesis of transmission via ruminant-derived protein meal. The use of ruminant-derived protein in sheep and cattle feeds was subsequently banned because of the plausibility of this hypothesis. In the case of an explosive outbreak, such as the sudden cattle feedlot deaths or IBD in village chickens, working hypotheses and initial corrective actions are needed within hours based on experience and first impressions. Formal analyses can be undertaken later to either confirm or refute initial impressions. For example, numerous sudden deaths in a feed lot with no apparent spatial pattern would initially suggest a common source epidemic so it could be useful to empty all the feed troughs and make sure water sources were clean and wholesome before proceeding further.

Intensive Follow-up

This includes clinical, pathological, microbiological and toxicological examinations as well as epidemiological analyses. Epidemiological follow-up will include detailed analysis of the data as well as the search for additional cases on other premises. Flow charts of management and movement of animals and feedstuffs may be required as part of this process. Feeding trials may be required where toxins are suspected as well as transmission experiments for possible infectious agents. In some cases intensive investigation of recent environmental and weather events will also be important.

Control and Prevention

Strategies to stop the epidemic must be put in place as soon as possible and will often be undertaken in the absence of conclusive findings. It may not be possible to stop an outbreak in a village once it starts but the detailed investigation of a number of outbreaks could provide valuable insight into possibly important 'component' causes.

Reporting

Finally, someone has to document the findings. For small outbreaks, this may take the form of a brief discussion with the farm manager outlining the important features and actions required to prevent future occurrences. However, it is wise to always produce some form of written report so that a permanent record of events exists for future use. For large outbreaks, findings should be published in the scientific literature. Gardner (1990) has outlined the essential features of a report on an outbreak investigation. For substantial investigations the report should contain the following sections: background, methods, results, hypotheses, financial impact (where appropriate), recommendations and appendices containing laboratory reports etc.

Surveillance and Monitoring

The term *surveillance* implies an active process in which data are collected, analysed, evaluated and reported to those involved with a goal of providing better control of a disease or condition. The term *monitoring* is usually used for a more passive process although in common usage both terms are often used interchangeably. Because of the substantial cost involved programs usually encompass several diseases at the one time. The term surveillance may be unacceptable politically because of the connotation of spying on individuals. Important questions that are often asked directly or indirectly as part of programs are:

- Is the frequency of the disease remaining constant, increasing or decreasing?
- What is the relative frequency of one disease compared with another?
- Are there differences in the geographical pattern of the condition?
- Does the disease have any impact on productivity and/or profitability?
- Is the disease absent from a particular herd, region, or nation?
- Is a control or eradication program cost-effective?

The data for surveillance programs may be generated by a number of methods which include clinical evaluations, laboratory reports, slaughter inspection data, screening tests, or owner reports. Surveillance programs may be developed at a number of different levels. Some examples are listed below.

Individual Farms: These usually include monitoring of economically significant variables to the individual, e.g. mortality, somatic cell count of milk, growth rate or milk production. The temporal pattern of these variables to identify potential problems is important.

Region or State: This may involve testing to establish freedom from particular diseases which may give individuals collective financial advantages over competitors, such as brucellosis freedom, or footrot protected areas.

National: Such programs are usually very costly if active. To help defray costs these programs may predominantly be based on owner-made diagnoses and involve testing of only a sample of the national herd. Passive surveillance schemes are in place in many countries for the early detection of foreign and/or emerging diseases. Such schemes often depend on recognition by livestock owners or veterinarians of suspicious disease signs.

Validity of Data

The validity of data is of primary concern when using field data for disease monitoring. For example, studies in the United States of America indicate that owners, and to a lesser extent veterinarians, are only able to categorise diseases into broad categories—for example, diarrhoea and pneumonia are usually not very sensitive or specific in the determination of the involvement of specific aetiologic agents. A recent study of preweaning mortality in pigs indicated that owners were only moderately sensitive but highly specific in identifying the cause of death among preweaned pigs. There were also marked differences among individual owners and with the age of the dead pig.

Surveillance systems should be designed to ensure that data of high quality be collected. Misclassification of disease status usually leads to an underestimation of the frequency of the condition and its economic impact. Moreover, if the misclassification is non-differential the odds ratio will be biased towards 1 in studies of risk factors for the disease in question.

Population at Risk

The biases described above affect numerator calculations but estimation of the population at risk is also important. Such denominators may be readily established on an individual farm but often become increasing more difficult to establish for state and national programs unless good data bases are available.

Monitoring based on Prevalence or Incidence Data

One of the main difficulties in recording incidence data is the necessity to maintain a continuous watch over the population to record new occurrences of disease. Prevalence is a poor substitute for incidence for diseases with high mortality or high case fatality rates. Incidence may, however, be estimated from repeated prevalence surveys of endemic disease.

Production and Disease Targets

An important component of production and disease monitoring is the setting of targets for important variables. Two important questions that should be considered are:

How many need to be monitored? How should targets be set for an individual herd? The following factors need to taken into consideration:

- the previous performance of the herd;
- comparable herds of the same size in the same area;
- where the owner would like to be in the future; and
- biological constraints.

For an exceptionally good herd, the goal may be to just maintain the herd's relative position or perhaps to redirect monitoring towards financial parameters including maintaining the same production level with fewer costs, e.g. reduce sow numbers by 10%. Specialised computer-based software is available to assist with monitoring many health and production parameters in dairy and swine herds but most have only limited ability to analyse data and identify problems. The ability to achieve a higher level of sophistication in the analysis usually requires a veterinarian with sound epidemiological skills.

Detecting Disease

The prevention of disease spread through the movement of live animals can be reduced by diagnostic testing and certification by appropriate authorities. For terrestrial animals such as cattle, serological tests are available for many diseases and every animal in a shipment may be tested. However, such a strategy may be impractical in some instances and only a sample of animals may be tested to decide if the group is infected or not with a certain level of confidence.

What is not commonly realised is that testing for disease at the group level incorporates a number of factors additional to those relevant to testing at the individual animal level. Thus, techniques such as serology which may be highly sensitive and specific at the individual animal level can still result in misclassification of a high proportion of groups where only a small proportion are tested.

At the individual animal level, diagnostic test performance is determined by its sensitivity and specificity. From an epidemiological perspective, sensitivity is the proportion of animals infected with the agent of interest which test positive while specificity is the proportion of uninfected animals which test negative. Additional factors which come into play when a group of animals is to be classified are the number of animals tested, the prevalence of disease in the group and the level of statistical confidence required that the group is truly negative. The only way to be 100% confident that no animals comprising a particular group are infected with a particular agent is to test every animal in the group with a diagnostic test which has perfect sensitivity and specificity. However, if only a low proportion of individual animals in the group are infected and only a small number are tested there can be quite a high chance that infected groups will be misclassified as uninfected.

The situation is further complicated where the diagnostic test being used has imperfect sensitivity and specificity which is the case for many of those in use in livestock. Table 2. The number of infected animals which can be in a group of 100 000 despite a sample testing negative using a test with perfect sensitivity and specificity at the individual animal level. No. of animals in sample tested from group of 100 000 and found negative. No. of infected animals which could be in the group despite the sample testing negative (two levels of confidence shown)

OIE International Animal Health Code

The codes of the Office International des Epizooties (OIE) form the basis for the establishment of international arrangements and dispute settlement with regard to quarantine issues in agricultural trade between among countries of the World Trade Organisation. For terrestial animals, the relevant code is the International Animal HealthCode, sometimes simply called 'the code'.

OIE Code—Surveillance

Expert consultations are used to assist in reviewing and developing codes. Any changes proposed by the relevant commissions must be ratified by member countries at an OIE general session. Through this process the OIE has developed international standards for surveillance for three diseases: BSE, rinderpest and contagious bovine pleuropneumonia.

The stated purpose of these standards is "to provide evidence that a country or region is free from disease or infection" and that "disease surveillance should be implemented by both: a system of reporting any signs of disease activity which come to the notice of Veterinary Services or livestock owners; and an active program of statistically-selected samples from host populations in order to detect clinical signs or other indications of the occurrence of the disease or transmission of infection."

In demonstrating that a country or zone is free of disease it will be necessary to conduct a surveillance program that would have a very high probability of detecting the disease if it were present. According to the contagious bovine pleuropneumonia guidelines, surveillance should include a combination of clinical, pathological, serological and microbiological methods based on an epidemiological approach. The mix of procedures will depend on the specific circumstances of the country or zone. It is therefore clear that the surveillance system will need to include both passive and active elements. The herd is the sampling unit. A sampling unit for the purposes of disease investigation and surveillance is defined as a group of animals in sufficiently close contact that individuals in the group would be at approximately equal risk of coming in contact with the disease agent if there were an infectious animal in the group. Under the OIE codes, disease surveillance activities must be conducted on populations stratified according to the management system and by herd size. Herds are to be selected by proper random statistical procedures for each stratum.

For both rinderpest and contagious bovine pleuropneumonia, the guidelines on serological surveillance suggest that sample sizes must be sufficient to provide a 95% probability of detecting evidence of the disease if it were present at a prevalence of 1% of herds. As the number of samples required will be affected by the sensitivity of the test used, the sample size must be adjusted to allow for any lack of sensitivity in the testing procedure. Cattle and any other susceptible domestic species *must be included* in the serosurveillance program. Wild susceptible species *must be sampled where possible* and domestic stock in contact with them *should be sampled intensively*.

OIE Code—Risk Analysis

Because of the potential impact of infectious diseases many countries are in the process of undertaking risk analyses to prevent the entry and spread of unwanted pathogens as trade in animal products increases under the various World Trade Organisation agreements. For example, in Australia a ban on the import of shrimp products not for human consumption was applied in November 1996. This was a direct result of the recent waves of infectious diseases which have occurred in farmed shrimp throughout the world and will be maintained until the results of a full import risk analysis are available.

The reason the ban applies to products not for human consumption is that these include bait for fishing as well as manufactured aquatic animal foodstuffs which will come in direct contact with populations of both wild and cultured shrimp. This is regarded as posing a high risk of introduction of diseases until the risks can be more carefully evaluated. The code on risk analysis contains new concepts to be embraced by animal disease control authorities. The code consists of four chapters: general considerations; guidelines for risk assessment; evaluation of veterinary services; and zoning and regionalisation of countries.

The principle of import risk analysis is to provide importing countries with an objective, defensible method of assessing the risks associated with the importation of animals, animal products, animal genetic material, feedstuffs, biological material and pathological material. The analysis should be transparent in order that the exporting country may be provided with a clear and substantiated decision on the conditions imposed for importation or refusal for importation. Following these principles is preferable to a zero-risk approach because it should lead to a more objective decision and enable competent authorities to discuss any differences in conclusion which may arise concerning potential risks.

The components of import risk analysis identified by the OIE include: *risk assessment* (identifying and estimating the risks and evaluating the consequences), *risk management* (identification, documentation and implementation of measures that can be used to reduce the risks and their consequences) and *risk communication* (means of communicating the results of the risk assessment to decision-makers, regulators, industry and the public); evaluation of *competent authorities*; within countries.

A standardised *risk assessment* method is prescribed in the code. The importing country should elaborate scenarios by which the introduction of a disease agent in an imported commodity and its subsequent exposure and transmission to animals is possible. Each scenario should comprise a set of factors that require identification (and quantification if possible) to allow estimation of risk.

Four categories of factors are identified: *country factors*—principally the prevalence of the disease agent in the population from which the commodity was drawn. *Commodity factors*—parameters specific to a particular commodity that affect the probability of disease agent presence and survival in a commodity at the time of import. *Exposure factors*—factors specific to the use and distribution of the commodity in the importing country which will affect the probability that a susceptible host species will be exposed and infected risk *reduction factors*—measures that can be applied to reduce the risk that a disease agent will be introduced into the importing country or exposed and/or transmitted to an animal.

For each of the above categories a number of options is identified in the code. In practice, information on each of the factors is obtained from available sources including precedents, scientific information, experience and expert opinion. Where possible, quantitative data are obtained for a factor. Where quantitative data is sparse or unreliable a qualitative risk assessment may be made.

Animal Health Information Systems

The international trading environment is changing. To remain competitive, both exporting and importing countries must anticipate and respond to these changes. The challenge will be to maintain an acceptable level of biosecurity while retaining access to export markets or protection from potentially 'risky' agricultural products.

Pressure for Better Information

There is a growing recognition among veterinary administrators throughout the world of the need for more quantitative and reliable information on livestock production and disease (Morris 1991). Better information is critical to efficient and effective disease control as well as becoming increasingly important in certification for international trade in livestock and livestock products. In developed countries, where production and health recording systems are now a key management tool in intensive animal industries, the issue is pertinent mainly to extensive grazing animal systems. Animal health information is required for a number of purposes including:

- international disease reporting obligations;
- public health and product certification;
- certification of livestock exports;
- international trade negotiations;
- management of national disease control programs; and
- priority-setting for research.

Animal disease reporting in the Asian and Pacific regions was the subject of a recent international workshop (Anon 1990a) and country review (Anon 1990b) jointly sponsored by the Asian Development Bank and the OIE. Findings from this project emphasised the universality and urgency of the need for improved animal health information in the region. The problem with many existing passive systems such as disease notification schemes and diagnostic laboratory records is that the basic data are frequently unrepresentative of the situation in the reference population (Ogundipe et al. 1989).

Overview of Animal Information Systems

There are a number of published overviews of animal information systems (Blajan 1979; Blood and Brightling 1988; OIE 1988, 1991) as well as specific regional examples (King 1985; Rolfe 1985; Doohoo 1988; Ogundipe et al. 1989; McKenzie and Thompson 1991; Martinez et al. 1992). Historically, information systems have serviced the need to record traditional government veterinary services of detecting disease outbreaks and assessing spread. Such systems keep account of activities and past progress rather than provide information on which to base decisions on future strategies. The need to rationally set priorities and identify the effectiveness of control strategies is gaining increasing importance with a concomitant recognition of the need for a variety of types of information depending on the particular purpose.

A good animal health information system should provide a reliable picture of the disease situation in a specified animal population. It should have a clear purpose and incorporate planned methods of data acquisition, management analysis and interpretation. In addition, desirable attributes are prompt reporting procedures and ongoing quality assurance (Morris 1991). There are a variety of sources of information on livestock production and diseases (Thrusfield 1995). These include compulsory notification schemes; saleyard and abattoir records; reports from routine and special investigations such as surveys and sentinel monitoring as well as laboratory records and targeted active surveillance.

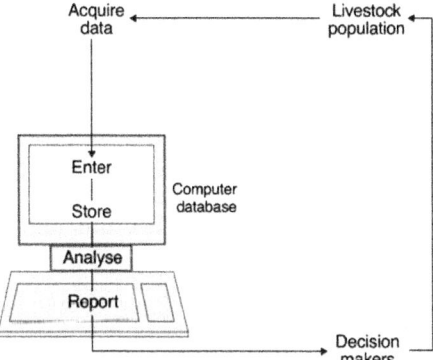

Figure 9: The general structure of an animal health information system and its relationships to data and decisions.

Conclusions

Developing good livestock disease surveillance systems means having capabilities in a range of areas. First, good disease investigation and diagnostic personnel and facilities are required to ensure reliable data are gathered. Second, there must be a good reason for collecting the data and the resultant reports must be useful in providing information on which sound decisions can be made. Finally, the communities likely to be affected by the decisions made as a result of animal health surveillance must be involved in the process and be provided with feedback.

Chapter 4

Economic Issues in Animal Health Programs

In a broad sense, the economic component of the Thai–Australia Animal Health Program has been concerned with generation of *information* on costs and benefits of animal health programs. More specifically, the economic research has focused in particular on the Thai control and eradication program against foot-and-mouth disease (FMD) in cattle, buffalo and swine. However, this has necessarily involved investigation of a variety of issues. Some of the specific areas which have been investigated include:

- the role of economics in animal health programs, including integrating economists into multidisciplinary animal health teams;
- the appropriate framework and methodology for economic analysis;
- estimation of costs of livestock diseases;
- the nature, extent and distribution of benefits from disease control and eradication;
- data needs, availability and validity for economic analysis;
- production systems and trade in Thai livestock industries; and
- the cost-effectiveness of various components of the Thai FMD control and eradication program, e.g. active surveillance of disease incidence, mass vaccination, and transport controls.

Some consideration has been given to other diseases in cattle, buffalo and pigs, as well as poultry diseases. In addition, a component of the research has focused on the value of information for animal health programs in Queensland, Australia. Within this broad context, a number of studies have been carried out to investigate particular aspects of Thai livestock industries and cost–benefit aspects of animal health programs. This paper will first examine conceptual and theoretical issues of economic analysis, then summarise the results of a number of particular economic studies. The material presented here draws on the series *Research Papers and Reports in Animal Health Economics*, published by the Department of Economics of The University of Queensland, which comprises over 40 papers produced during the Australian Centre for International Agricultural Research (ACIAR) project.

The Role and Methods of Economic Analysis in Animal Health

In general, economic analysis is designed to provide decision-support information for government and private agents involved in livestock industries. Such information increases knowledge of the economic trade-offs involved when particular policies are adopted. The analysis takes an anthropocentric approach in that alternative policies are evaluated in terms of costs and benefits to humans (producers, consumers, traders, government). In general, a social cost–benefit framework is adopted in which the economic criterion applied is 'willingness-to-pay', which can be measured in terms of producer and consumer 'profit' or *economic surplus*. In a multidisciplinary project such as the Thai–Australian Animal Health Project, economic analysis relates to and draws on technical information on livestock production and disease impact parameters, so that costs and returns to the various stakeholder groups can be examined. The economic analysis can only be as reliable as the technical information on which it is based, although sensitivity analysis can be applied to determine the impact of varying parameter estimates.

Economic evaluation of national animal health programs requires analysis from the producer level through to the national level and the inclusion of trade impacts. To the extent possible, cost and benefit categories should include both direct and immediate changes in livestock production as well as long-term changes in herd structure and genetic quality, ability to intensify production, and non-market impacts such as those relating to animal welfare and the environment.

Development and Adaptation of Economic Theory to Animal Health Issues

A relatively small number of economists have expert skills in economic analysis of animal health programs, and economic evaluation frameworks used for their work remain controversial. Hence it has been necessary to consider appropriate evaluation methods for the particular issues examined.

Optimal Disease Control Effort

The social cost–benefit analysis (CBA) framework generally accepted for evaluation of animal health programs involves making estimates of all socially relevant costs and benefits, including both market and non-market items, and hence deriving 'incremental cash flows' for the 'with control' and 'without control' situations. From these, discounted cash flow performance criteria such as benefit-to-cost (B:C) ratios, net present value (NPV) and internal rate of return (IRR) can be derived. In practice, difficulties can arise in interpreting these criteria.

When expenditure levels vary, the NPV may not rank alternative animal health programs correctly. One program with a slightly higher NPV than another may involve substantially greater expenditure, hence the rate of return on investment may be lower. Under particular cash flow patterns, the IRR can be non-existent, non-unique or perverse (increasing as the cost of capital increases).

Also, it has been demonstrated that the comparison of B:C ratios for alternative disease control programs could lead to an inferior choice (McInerney 1991). A control program involving a relatively small expenditure could have a higher B:C ratio than a more ambitious program, yet the program involving the greater expenditure could result in greater overall benefits.

In an attempt to define optimal expenditure on animal health more clearly, a graphical exposition involving a loss–expenditure tradeoff curve has been developed (McInerney 1988, 1991; McInerney et al. 1992). This takes the form of a concave tradeoff curve between disease cost (C) and control expenditure (E) as illustrated. The points along this *loss– expenditure frontier* may be taken to represent the capitalised value, or discounted sum, of disease and expenditure costs over a number of years.

This curve represents the choice set available to a country in terms of effort on disease control. With no control expenditure, there is a high disease cost $c1$. As control expenditure is increased, disease cost first decreases rapidly, the C–E tradeoff curve being almost vertical, but with increasing expenditure the curve flattens as the marginal rate of improvement with respect to cost declines.

If the disease can be eradicated, control expenditure may fall to zero or to some low amount representing the cost of preventing new outbreaks.

Since both axes are expressed in dollar terms, and a dollar in disease cost is regarded as equivalent to a dollar in control costs, the line with slope −1 represents combinations of equal cost to the country, i.e. an *isocost line*. One such line is drawn; this is the line which is tangent to the C–E curve. Any C–E combination to the right of this line would represent greater overall cost while any point to the left is not achievable.

Hence e^* is the Economic Issues in Animal Health Programs 61optimal expenditure level and is associated with a disease cost c^* (total cost. For this formulation, the disease cost variable would need to embrace all relevant items including non-market costs (e.g. environmental impacts, animal welfare changes).

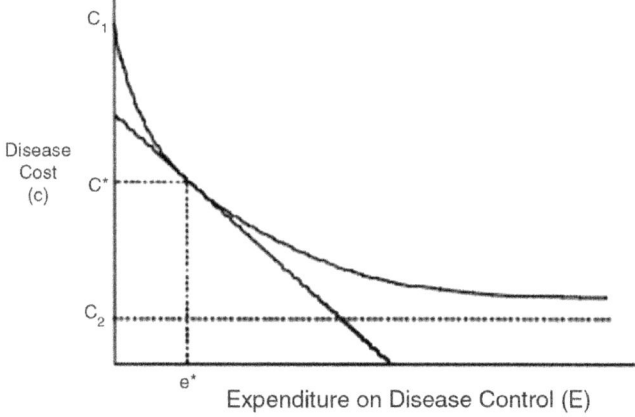

Figure 1: The McInerney loss-expenditure trade-off model

The McInerney model has two important limitations. The first concerns setup costs such as construction of a vaccine production plant, recruiting staff, and public awareness programs, all of which impose overhead costs before any control activities can be conducted in the field. The kinked nature of the C–E curve results in the optimal control expenditure being much greater in relative terms than in Figure earlier. A moderate level of control expenditure such as $e1$ results in the worst of both worlds, namely substantial control expenditure and little or no reduction of disease costs.

Figure also reveals that the option of zero control expenditure may be superior to most of the possible expenditure levels on the C–E tradeoff curve. In fact, the disease cost when there is no control expenditure would only have to fall by a small amount to be on a lower isocost line that the point identified as optimal.

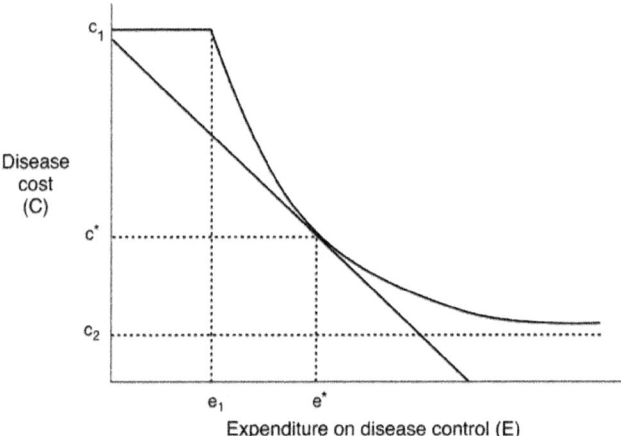

Figure 2: Disease cost–control expenditure trade-off model for an infectious disease.

The second limitation of the McInerney model is that, particularly in the case of infectious diseases, a low level of control activity may be ineffective in preventing disease spread. For example, a 20% or even 50% vaccination coverage for FMD may protect the vaccinated animals but would not be sufficient to make substantial progress towards eradication. When most animals are protected, it becomes possible to eradicate the disease from the population. The major gains from disease eradication are:

- production losses are avoided;
- if the disease is trade-limiting, new markets may be opened up and a price increase achieved; and
- expenditure may no longer be incurred on control.

While the first of these will not change much from a low incidence of the disease to eradication, major gains in trade and reduced control expenditure are not likely to arise until a disease is totally eradicated. This would probably be the case with FMD, where new export markets can be expected to become available only when international recognition of disease-free status is achieved.

These considerations suggest that the McInerney model may only be appropriate for localised diseases for which control programs have low overhead costs, such as mastitis in dairy cattle. That is, it is applicable to special cases of disease control only and *"is not justified in the context of economic decisions about the control of different livestock diseases"* (Tisdell 1995, p. 21). The dichotomous choice situation of mentioned Figure contrasts strongly with the conclusion of McInerney (1991, p. 152) with respect to disease eradication programs, of *"the importance of identifying the full loss–* expenditure relationship for economic analysis rather than hiding behind the *apparent neatness of the CBA technique".* In fact, where the loss–expenditure curve is concave, the conclusion of McInerney (1991) that benefit–cost ratios fail to rank alternatives correctly would not hold.

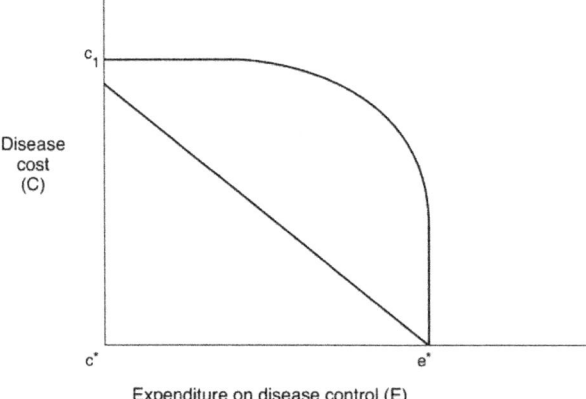

Figure 3: Disease cost–control expenditure tradeoff model for an infectious disease which requires a threshold protection level.

Distribution of Benefits for Disease Control Programs

Another area of theoretical modelling has been extension of stakeholder analysis to include not only producer benefits, but also impacts on traders and consumers of livestock products, government fiscal impacts, and trade gains from expanded foreign markets.

The Value of Animal Health Information to Decision-makers

Epidemiological modelling and Bayesian decision theory have been combined as a methodology for estimating the value to landholders of additional information on animal health. The application of this research in a Queensland context is reported in Ramsay et al. (1997c) and in Chapter 14 of this book.

Application of Cost–benefit Analysis to Animal Health Programs

An investigation has been made of the methodological issues and practical difficulties of applying social CBA to animal health programs. This arose out of the CBA component of a workshop for veterinary epidemiologists which took place in Lampang, Thailand, in January 1995, and is documented in Harrison (1996a).

Availability and Collection of Disease Incidence Data

Any economic analysis of animal health programs requires reliable data on disease incidence. This raises questions of how to collect these data in a costeffective manner, and how reliable these data are.

Disease Inder-reporting in Passive Reporting Systems

There is strong anecdotal and research evidence of under-reporting of the incidence of livestock diseases, which can present difficulties in economic evaluation of disease control programs. Typically, reporting follows a sequence of steps, from the individual producers, through veterinary officers, to regional and national recording bureaus, and to international agencies. There are thus many stages at which under-reporting can occur. A landmark study in under-reporting of disease cases is that of Ogundipe et al. (1989) for Nigeria. According to these authors (p. 126): "*It is generally* known that many diseases occur, especially in rural areas, which are never *reported to veterinary authorities*" and outbreaks that are reported are "*no more than the tip of the iceberg*".

They found the animal disease reporting system in Nigeria is characterised by "*late, inaccurate and gross under reporting*". As an example, for Newcastle disease it was not possible to Economic Issues in Animal Health Programs 65estimate the rate of reporting from livestock owner to veterinary clinician, but at subsequent stages of reporting less than 20% of actual cases were reported for the period 1977 to 1984.

In case this be considered a problem confined to developing countries, mention may be made of the study by McCallon and Beal (1982) for the United States of America. These authors noted gross under-reporting of chorioptic cattle mange, where one small state (Vermont) disclosed four times as many cases of the disease as the other 49 states combined simply because there were trained people checking for the disease in that state.

Notification efficiency in the case of FMD in developing countries is probably quite poor. An early assessment of FMD reporting in Thailand made the observation that: "*The number of reported outbreaks is not identical with the* actual number of outbreaks. There exists the opinion, that only a few percent of *outbreaks are being reported*" (von Kreudener 1985, p. 126–127). Subsequently, Chaisrisongkram (1993, p. 25) noted that data collection methods used in the past were "*quite limited and not well suited to the need for control measures*". According to Ellis (1993, p. 58):*Official records of FMD incidence vary widely in quality. The disease may be somild where it is endemic that farmers may not recognise it and even if they dorecognise it they may not bother to report cases. Effects are usually transient* and insidious but often affect a large proportion of animals in the herd or flock.

It would be expected that the notification efficiency for FMD in Thailand would increase over time and that under-reporting is not as serious an issue now with improved communications, better equipped veterinary officers and greater financial commitment to FMD eradication. Of course, the difficulty still arises in that livestock owners may not recognise mild FMD cases, or may not report cases. Where 'stamping out' (slaughter of infected animals) is a possibility, and livestock owners believe they will not be fully compensated for slaughtered animals, there would be an incentive for not reporting cases. Discussions with various veterinary experts suggest that the current notification efficiency for FMD in Thailand is of the order of 5% to 20%.

Cost-effective Survey Designs for Active Surveillance

Taking blood samples from large animals and subjecting these to laboratory analysis for titres against FMD is a highly expensive process; hence a sampling design which provides the most reliable information for a given expenditure is required. Typically, a two-stage probability proportional to size (PPS) sampling design is employed in which a sample of villages is 66 Animal Health in Southeast Asia chosen and then livestock are chosen from selected villages. The specific sampling design for a given budget, or accuracy target, will depend on a number of estimated parameters for the reference livestock population and cost parameters for each stage of sampling. The statistical theory underlying PPS sampling is highly complex, and collaboration with the Queensland Government Statistician's Office was obtained in this work.

The World Health Organisation recommended design, consisting of 30 villages and seven subjects from each, was found to be quite robust with respect to variations in population protection status and sampling cost parameters. In active surveillance for FMD (tests of seroprevalence), there was a tendency for 'natural' optima to arise with respect to sampling designs, due to cost discontinuities, such as where a maximum number of blood specimens can be collected per day (Harrison 1996b). Details of sampling designs relevant to active surveillance for FMD protection in northern Thailand are discussed in Chapter 8 of this book.

Findings from Specific Applications Thai Livestock Industry Studies

Data have been collected from various sources to develop profiles of livestock industries in Thailand as a background to investigating production benefits and trade opportunities from improved animal health (Murphy and Tisdell 1995a–c, 1996; Kehren and Tisdell 1997a; Smith and Harrison 1997). Reports have been prepared for the meat cattle and buffalo, dairy, pig and poultry industries. These reports have examined livestock numbers, management systems and disease status. Unlike cattle and buffalo, the pig and poultry industries have clearly defined commercial and village sectors, and disease control in the latter presents considerable difficulty. The highly cyclical nature of village pig production associated with pigmeat prices militates against regular vaccination for FMD.

Socioeconomic and Environmental Studies

The success of any livestock disease control program will depend on the feasibility and willingness of livestock owners to cooperate with the program. In Thailand, small-scale ownership of cattle, buffalo and pigs means that important decisions concerning disease reporting, vaccination, livestock movements and so on are made within the village socioeconomic environment. Securing producer cooperation is more difficult than for commercial pig and dairy holdings, where disease costs are more apparent Economic Issues in Animal Health Programs 67and ability to afford control measures is greater. Cross-sectional survey data from Thai villages have been used in socioeconomic analysis of the role of Livestock in villages (Murphy and Tisdell 1995d).

It has been found that consideration needs to be given to the role of women and of common property resources in the management of Thai village livestock production systems (Kehren and Tisdell 1996). While livestock production is a form of value-adding relative to crop production, the efficiency with which human nutritional wants are met is lower, and this can lead to greater adverse environmental impacts (Tisdell and Harrison 1997).

FMD Global Status and Incidence in Thailand

A review has been undertaken of the global status of foot-and-mouth disease in bovines. The prevalence of this disease in Asia and the need for a coordinated control program is notable (Murphy 1996). Statistics on FMD incidence from various sources, including Thai researchers and government agencies and the Office International des

Epizooties (OIE), have been summarised and interpreted in an attempt to gain an understanding of the importance of this disease in Thai livestock industries (Kehren and Tisdell 1997b).

The Role of Animal Health in Economic Development

The costs of livestock diseases and the benefits of disease control have been examined in the context of national economic development, with particular reference to Thailand (Harrison and Tisdell 1997).

Macroeconomic Analysis of Livestock Industries

A closed general equilibrium (CGE) model was applied to examine the relationship between output of the livestock sector (as influenced by disease control measures) and other Thai industries (Purcell et al. 1997).

Collaboration in Studies Conducted Through Chiang Mai University

Two collaborative projects were established at the University of Chiang Mai, in the Departments of Agricultural Economics and Livestock Science and the Multiple Cropping Unit. These studies involved a survey of village livestock producers in Chiang Mai province (Thani et al. 1997), and an intensive survey of animal health in dairy production. Dairy production was found to consist of small herds, in which comprehensive vaccination programs typically are adopted.

Cost–benefit Aspects of the Thai FMD Control and Eradication Program

This analysis (S.R. Harrison and C.A. Tisdell, unpublished data) integrates findings of other components of the project to estimate the social payoff from the current Thai FMD control and eradication program. Although major data problems arose, the analysis provides indicative results that the program has a positive net present value and a benefit–cost ratio exceeding unity. However, it is doubtful that the rate of return on public funds is nearly as high as estimated in an earlier evaluation by Bartholomew and Culpitt (in 1992).

The producer benefits appear to be smaller than would be anticipated for FMD eradication from an European perspective. As well, the potential for increased livestock and meat exports from Thailand as a result of FMD eradication appears rather limited. However, provided current control measures are continued and adapted as necessary, the Thai FMD program appears to be well justified when all categories of benefits (including reduced animal health expenditure, trade gains, transport and draught, and animal welfare benefits) are taken into account. The importance of FMD eradication in Thailand becomes greater when viewed within a program of eradication in Southeast Asia. Such a program may take several decades to achieve its goal.

Difficulties Encountered and Lessons from the Project

From the viewpoint of the economics component, the Thai–Australia Animal Health Project faced a number of difficulties. While a project such as this would not be expected to be all 'plain sailing', and language difficulties and data scarcity are inevitable, the difficulties were somewhat greater than anticipated. Important amongst these were:

- delay in signing the memorandum of understanding in Thailand, thus reducing the effective project duration;
- difficulties in communication between disciplines, demonstrating the need for cross-disciplinary training with immersion into the disciplines;
- lack of biological data on FMD impacts (e.g. mortality and reproduction rates and extent of compensatory weight gains) in the village livestock sector where the disease is endemic;
- absence of staff in Thai livestock agencies with economics training, and hence a lack of understanding of the data needs for economic analysis;
- political sensitivity in Thailand about animal health issues, and unwillingness to disclose information about livestock disease incidence and expenditure on animal health programs; and
- unavailability of Thai postgraduate agricultural economics students to participate in field work in Thailand, the early termination of some of the data collection activities in Thailand, and restricted access to survey data.

Persistent efforts at data collection were continued and, given the circumstances, it is considered that reasonably representative data were obtained for economic assessment purposes.

Concluding Comments

Economic analysis has been applied to a number of issues in the Thai– Australia Animal Health Program to aid understanding of disease control options and their cost and benefit implications for the various stakeholder groups. While major problems with data shortage exist, considerable insights have been gained into the appropriateness of disease control measures.

Disease Focus : Foot-and-mouth Disease

Foot-and-mouth Disease

There are four vesicular diseases of pigs which are difficult or impossible to differentiate clinically: FMD, swine vesicular disease (SVD), vesicular exanthema (VES), and vesicular stomatitis (VS). Of these, FMD is the most widespread and important with SVD being of secondary importance in some regions (e.g. the EU). The other two have very limited distribution and VES has disappeared.

Importance of FMD

FMD is the most important restraint to international trade in animals and animal products. Consequently, large sums of money have been invested in control and eradication programmes and also into research. As a result more is known about the FMD virus than about almost any other animal infection.

It generally produces severe disease in pigs and cattle.

FMD is so important because it is highly infectious, spreads rapidly throughout animal populations and over long distances on the wind and hence it is difficult and costly to control. Also because of its damaging and debilitating effect on cattle, a great deal of effort and tax-payers money has been spent keeping it out of large areas of the world. It would be highly irresponsible to let it back in.

If you live in an FMD-fringe area that is also free of swine vesicular disease (SVD) you should be aware of what early clinical signs would make you suspicious and what you should do if you suspected them in your herd. If you farm in an endemic area or a fringe area in which SVD is present then you should know a bit more, particularly about the clinical signs in pigs and vaccination regimes.

If you farm in an FMD-free country that takes sound precautions against its entry, the risk to your herd is negligible unless you farm in California where vesicular exanthema may pose a very small risk.

Susceptible Animals

Among farm animals, pigs, cattle, sheep, goats and deer are susceptible. In addition, wild and domestic cloven hooved animals such as hedgehogs and rats are also susceptible as are elephants.

Early Clinical Signs

In cattle the early clinical signs are much more definitive or suggestive than in pigs. For example in a dairy herd several cows may suddenly show depressed milk yield, go off their feed, run a fever, have a dramatic drop in milk yield, and a little later start salivating profusely, the saliva running from their mouths (slavering). If you see such signs, jump into action, ring the vet. Veterinarians who have to deal with FMD say that if a farmer telephones to say that several cows are salivating profusely they think first "FMD?".

If after cows have started salivating and smacking lips, vesicles are noticed on the lips, on the teats and around the coronets, the areas above hooves - your worst fears are probably true. The probability is that your pig herd has been infected too.

In pigs early signs are lameness a drop in food consumption and some pigs appear depressed and have fevers of about 40.5°C,(105°F). In piglets sudden death due to cardiac failure is common. What should make you strongly suspicious is the appearance a little later of vesicles up to 30mm. diametre, similar to those described above for cattle. They are most plentiful around the coronets but are less plentiful on the nose and lips although this is where you are likely to see them first. They often appear on the teats of recently farrowed sows. By then the sows and some of the other pigs may be dribbling saliva and chomping their jaws. If they are on bedding they may not appear lame but if they are on concrete they probably will be.

The early signs of swine vesicular disease (SVD) when it is severe, are indistinguishable from FMD so you should suspect it too.

If you farm near the coast of California where FMD and SVD are extremely unlikely, vesicular exanthema could be a possibility. If you farm in Georgia, the Carolinas or Central or South America and it is summer/autumn time perhaps you should think of vesicular stomatitis. The clinical signs of all four diseases are almost indistinguishable.

Within 24 hours many of the vesicles will have burst. On the lips and teats they may leave shallow erosions but on the coronets of the feet secondary infection and trauma may convert them into raw jagged-edged ulcers.

If the pigs are not killed some may lose their complete hooves (so-called "Thimbling"), sows may abort, as a result of fever, and in severe outbreaks some may die. Boars may go lame and stop serving sows, so there is an infertility side effect. There may also be an increase in mortality among suckled piglets. This is often the first sign.

In endemic areas where vaccination is carried out routinely the disease is not a serious economic problem in pig herds. In fringe areas, particularly where vaccination is not allowed (e.g. in the EU) it is a serious problem because the herd will almost certainly be slaughtered out and although compensation is likely to be paid, the farm cannot be restocked for at least six weeks, it is therefore out of production and in a negative cash flow for a long time.

Diagnosis

Rapid accurate diagnosis is essential.

FMD cannot be distinguished from SVD on clinical grounds, or from VES in California, although SVD is often much milder. To differentiate these diseases and confirm the presumptive diagnosis, samples have to be sent to a laboratory capable of making a diagnosis.

There are not many of these. The main one is the World Reference Laboratory at Pirbright near London in England. There is also one on Plum Island off the coast of NY in the USA and one near Melbourne in Australia.

The samples sent are blood and pieces of the skin that overlay the blisters plus vesicular fluid if this is available. Once the samples have been received by the laboratory diagnosis is fairly rapid.

Tests called ELISAs are used for virus identification and if it is FMD they also indicate what serotype it is. The virus may also be grown in cell culture and the identification confirmed by other tests. A molecular genetic test called a PCR (polymerase chain reaction) may also be used to 'fingerprint" the virus. The gene (genome or RNA) of FMD repeatedly undergoes minor changes as the virus spreads through animal populations so by identifying the precise sequence in the gene the laboratory staff are able to make an assumption where it may have come from by the most recent isolate with a similar sequence.

Treatment

- There is no treatment. Animals should be destroyed.

Management Control and Prevention

Vaccination (where applicable):

- In endemic and high risk areas routine vaccination may be practised mainly to protect the breeding stock.

- Most FMD vaccines are produced in cell suspension cultures and inactivated by ethylenamine derivatives. An adjuvant is added to make them more potent. Oily adjuvants are used in swine.

- Vaccination in pigs is problematical. This is because protection is short-lived lasting only about six months. It is also partly because there are seven serotypes of FMD and protection against one leaves animals susceptible to the others. Vaccines must be multivalent (several serotypes) in most endemic regions. Since FMD is largely a winter disease, vaccination should be carried out in the autumn.

- Serotypes - There are 7 main serotypes: A, O, C, SAT 1, SAT 2, SAT 3 and Asia 1. There are also many strains within serotypes. Careful selection of the strains for incorporation in vaccines is essential to ensure they are effective.

Precautions

- Countries in free and fringe areas apply strictly enforced national preventative measures against the introduction of infection. The main features of these measures are control over the importation of cloven-hoofed animals and of meat from such animals from counties in which FMD occurs.

- The virus does not survive rigor mortis but it can persist in bone marrow and lymph nodes of infected carcasses for several weeks.

- If the disease does enter a free or fringe area, a slaughter policy is implemented, all diseased and in-contact animals being slaughtered. A standstill on animal movement is imposed and tracings are carried out to check possible spread of the disease through previous contacts. Ring vaccination may be used around the affected region.

- If you farm in an FMD-risk region you should take strict precautions against the contamination of your herd. If you have a cattle or goat herd or a flock of sheep as well as a pig herd you should also adopt preventative measures for them and keep a wary eye for the appearance of typical clinical signs.

- Unfortunately, none of the measures described prevent the windborne spread of FMD. Infected pigs can produce huge quantities of infective virus as aerosols. They produce far more aerosol virus than cattle, goats or sheep. In dry weather when there are strong thermals the aerosol virus is rapidly inactivated so the wind does not carry infective aerosols very far. Strong winds, hills and objects such as high buildings and trees create turbulence and disperse the plume of airborne virus as they would a plume of smoke from a bonfire. In humid overcast weather with a steady light wind blowing over flat countryside infective virus may survive long enough to infect other herds up to 60km (36 miles) distant. Over water, given the same climatic conditions, infective virus has been shown to travel up to 300km (180 miles) so siting your pig herd on an island in a lake is not going to stop it. Windborne infection is impossible to guard against. Even if your pig herd is in closed buildings, the aerosol virus can get in through the ventilation system and you may carry it in from outside on your boots or clothes.

- If vaccination is permitted and the pig herd is in a high-risk area you should consider routine vaccination to reduce the susceptibility of your herd.

Basic Biosecurity

Basic biosecurity measures are important in helping to minimise the spread of disease, and this becomes critical when there is a high risk of infection from a specific disease outbreak. These measures are important, unfortunately foot and mouth can spread on the wind and is therefore that much more difficult to keep out, however the following procedures could help to reduce the risk.

Biosecurity Measures

1. Standardise pig movements and keep to an absolute minimum.
2. People and Vehicles are a potential source of potential contamination.
3. Only allow essential visitors on to the farm and provide your own boots and clothing at the entrance.
4. If visitors do not shower ensure hands are washed.
5. Limit the movement of people between buildings as much as possible.
6. Place foot dips at all entrances, service and feed delivery points. Use an approved disinfectant at the correct dilution.

7. Review all cleaning and disinfection procedures. Only allow cleaned and disinfected vehicles to visit your farm.

8. Adopt special precautions at loading ramps. Provide designated boots and overalls for use on the loading ramp only. Disinfect all loading areas before and after use. Check drainage is away from the farm.

9. Clean all pens thoroughly. These should be disinfected and dried between pig groups.

Using the following protocol for cleaning swine facilities:

1. Soften dirt and manure in heavily soiled areas using a low-pressure water spray. Leave to soak for a few hours.

2. Once softened, use high-pressure sprays (750 psi to 2,000 psi preferred) to remove all the dirt and organic material.

   o Start at the back of the pen or building and work toward the front.

   o Spray the ceiling first, then the walls and finally the floor.

   o Use sprayers and nozzles that allow you to wash hard-to-reach areas, including the undersides of troughs, feeders and flooring when possible.

3. Once the pen is clean, rinse all surfaces to remove accumulated aerosol organic material.

4. Spray on surfactant or emulsifying agent to remove any residual organic materials.

5. Rinse all surfaces.

6. Thoroughly Disinfect (NOTE: Disinfectants only work on clean surfaces).

   o Disinfectants work best at temperatures above 65° F, but not above 110° F.

   o Follow the manufacturer's application instructions for the product.

   o Apply the disinfectant with pressure (ideally through pressure washer) to force disinfectant into pores, cracks and crevices. Fog or aerosol application is a second alternative.

   o Move from back to front and from top to bottom of the room.

7. Allow the building time to dry.

8. Leave rooms vacant for as long as the production system will allow before repopulating.

How to Protect your Farm?

This leaflet provides information on preventative measures on how to protect your farm against foot and mouth disease. Further measures apply if your farm is in a declared infected area.

The following measures should be followed:

- You should ensure you maintain the highest standards of hygiene for all movements on and off your farm.

- Have only one combined entrance and exit. Display the name of the farm and the telephone number on the gate. Keep the gate locked.

- Provide a means of contact between farm entrance and house for essential callers, e.g. a bell or a gong. Supply a tub of disinfectant, a brush for scrubbing footwear and a spray pump. Keep the disinfectant solution clean and renew it daily.

- All vehicles entering and leaving the premises should have their wheels sprayed with approved disinfectant.

- Stop all non-essential vehicles and visitors from entering the farm and arrange whenever possible for collection and delivery of supplies to take place at farm boundary.

- Keep a record of all deliveries. In the event of disease being confirmed this may help in epidemiological investigations.

- Where possible, house all the animals or keep them away from the perimetre of your farm.

- Ensure you complete all records of stock movements as required by existing legislation.

- Each farm must be treated as a separate unit. Make separate arrangements for labour, management and feeding.

- Keep dogs, cats and poultry under control.

- Make every effort to destroy rats and other vermin. They may spread the disease.

- Keep your stock away from household waste, bones or swill.

- Limit contact with other peoples livestock and with other keepers of livestock.

- Should you have any contact with them, before you go near your own animals, disinfect your footwear, change your clothes and wash with hot water and soap, including your hair. Any item or object that may have had contact with disease must also be disinfected.
- Healthcare officials are aware of precautions necessary and you must not delay seeking medical assistance if needed.

Disenfection

A dirty surface must be cleaned before it can be satisfactorily disinfected. The dirt may make the disinfectant useless. It is therefore most important that anything which must be disinfected is first soaked with an approved disinfectant, then thoroughly washed and cleaned and finally washed down with an approved disinfectant.

An Overview of the Disease from Defra

Early Notification

- Controlling the disease depends on the prompt reporting of all suspected cases. Delay allows the disease to get a start that is very difficult to overtake.
- Stock owners should therefore be constantly on the watch for any suspicious signs among their animals, even when the country is free from outbreaks of the disease.
- Special care is necessary with sheep and pigs where lameness is often the only sign. It must be remembered that animals can go lame for various reasons, of which foot and mouth disease could be one.
- Sheep lame apparently for another reason (for example foot rot) may also be affected by foot and mouth.
- Owners of livestock should always be suspicious when one or more animals become lame suddenly and the lameness becomes widespread in other animals on the premises.
- The owner of a suspected animal or carcase must by law notify the fact to the MAFF Divisional Veterinary Manager or to the police. The owner is not expected to diagnose the disease, but he ought to know enough about the disease to suspect it.
- All owners and stockmen should make themselves familiar with the signs, and call in a veterinary surgeon as early as

possible; they should never ask another stock-owner to look at the suspected animal.

- If the suspicion is strong it is better to notify as above without seeking other advice. If notification is via the police, they will at once get in touch with the Ministry's Divisional Veterinary Manager for the area who will immediately arrange, without cost to the owner, for the examination of the suspected animal. The Ministry's veterinary staff are available at all times, and if you suspect disease you are required to notify this suspicion immediately.

Clinical Signs

The interval between exposure to infection and the appearance of symptoms varies between twenty-four hours and ten days, or even longer. The average time is three to six days.

Cattle

- Slobbering and smacking lips.
- Shivering.
- Tender and sore feet.
- Reduced milk yield.
- Sores and blisters on feet.
- Raised temperature.

Sheep

- Sudden, severe lameness.
- Lies down frequently and is very unwilling to rise.
- When made to rise stands in a half-crouching position, with hind legs brought well forward, reluctant to move.
- Blisters may be found on the hoof where the horn joins the skin which may extend all round the coronet and in the cleft of the foot. When they burst the horn is separated from the tissues underneath, and hair round the hoof may appear damp.
- Blisters in the mouth are not always apparent but, when they do develop, form on the dental pad and sometimes the tongue.

Pigs

- Sudden lameness.
- Prefers to lie down.

- When made to move squeals loudly and hobbles painfully.
- Blisters form on the upper edge of the hoof, where the skin and horn meet, and on the heels and in the cleft.
- May extend right round the top of the hoof with the result that the horn becomes separated.
- Blisters may develop on the snout or on the tongue.
- It is important to remember that Swine Vesicular Disease has identical symptoms to foot-and-mouth disease. Therefore anyone who sees blisters in pigs must report the sighting as suspected foot-and-mouth disease until laboratory tests prove otherwise.

Spread

- Foot-and-mouth disease is extremely infectious. A very small quantity of the virus is capable of infecting an animal, and the disease could spread throughout the country if no attempt were made to control it.
- Airborne spread of the virus can take place and under favourable climatic conditions the disease may be spread considerable distances by this route.
- The virus is present in great quantity in the fluid from the blisters, and it can also occur in the saliva, exhaled air, milk and dung. Any of these can be a source of infection to other stock. At the height of the disease, virus is present in the blood and all parts of the body.
- Heat, sunlight and disinfectants will destroy the virus, whereas cold and darkness tend to keep it alive. Under favourable conditions it can survive for long periods.
- Animals pick up the virus either by direct or indirect (airborne) contact with an infected animal, or by contact with foodstuffs or other things which have been contaminated by such an animal, or by eating or coming into contact with some part of an infected carcase.
- Cattle trucks, lorries, market places, and loading ramps - where infected animals may have been present - are sources of infection until disinfected. Roads may also become contaminated, and virus may be picked up and carried on the wheels of passing vehicles such as delivery lorries, milk tankers etc.

- Any person who has attended diseased animals can spread the disease; and dogs, cats, poultry, wild game and vermin may also carry infected material.
- Previous outbreaks occurred in the eastern and south-eastern counties when the disease had been prevalent on the continent of Europe. In these cases infection was apparently brought to this country by airborne carriage of the virus under favourable climatic conditions. Imported meat, if found to be infected with the virus, may also be a source of infection.

Control

- All affected stock and any others which have been exposed to a risk of infection such that it is reasonably certain that they would develop the disease if left alive, are slaughtered. Full compensation is paid for animals slaughtered.
- MAFF supervise disinfection of the infected premises takes place, and no fresh stock can introduced without MAFF approval. In addition to this, the SVS imposes restrictions on the movement of animals within and into an infected area which extends for a radius of not less than 10 kilometres around the infected place, and no movement of animals into or out of this area is permitted.

Prevention and Treatment of Diseases—Some Methods

Treatment, or therapy, of disease may be defined as any effort to cure disease, arrest its course, lessen its severity, or alleviate the pain and inconvenience that disease causes. It includes the administration of drugs or medicines; physical therapy, such as massage, exercise, immobilisation with bandages or splints, and application of heat or cold; and any changes in methods of feeding or handling that are made to insure recovery.

Drug and physical treatments are sometimes called direct therapy; good management may be called indirect or supporting therapy.

The art of treating disease is as old as the history of man. Written records of some of the early civilizations describe some of the diseases of domestic animals and give directions for treating them. It is an art that has never stood still. Man has constantly striven to find better methods of restoring his sick animals to good health.

The use of drugs and medicines, including biological products such as vaccines and serums, constitute the most important segment of disease treatment. Until about 70 years ago, progress in developing new and better drug treatments was rather slow because the nature of disease was not well understood and a real scientific approach to treatment therefore was impossible, and because few organised, extensive efforts to find new treatments were being made.

The improvements that were taking place were coming largely from the trial-and-error experience of practicing veterinarians. A rapid development of experimental methods of studying both the normal and the sick animal began about 70 years ago. Such studies have added enormously to our knowledge of the science of disease.

We know now that many of the treatments used in the past were aimed at the results of disease rather than at disease itself. For example, we used to see animals (and people) treated for fever. Now it is generally recognised that fever may be brought on by many different causes. The skillful veterinarian of today tries to find out what is causing the fever and then treats the disease itself. Fever medicines, which were so generally used in the early years of this century, are seldom heard of now.

Experimental studies of the action of drugs have accompanied the studies of normal and sick animals. Physiologists and pharmacologists have measured and recorded the effects of a large number of drugs and medicines on animals kept under controlled conditions. We now know rather definitely what results may be expected from the use of many of the different remedies. We know, too, that many of the remedies in common use 70 years ago have little actual effect. Furthermore, some of the treatments that were formerly in rather general use are actually harmful. For example, carbolic acid (phenol), which was used to treat wounds, did so much damage to the tissues that its use actually slowed down healing.

Experimental studies have proved that the different species of animals may respond differently to the same drug. Thus dogs are put to sleep by morphine, but morphine causes cats to become restless and excited. Chloroform is a fairly safe anesthetic for the horse but a dangerous one for the hog. Dogs may be anesthetized with ether rather easily, but cows cannot be.

All these developments have given the veterinarian and the livestock owner a good foundation for a scientific approach to treatment of disease. With a fairly good understanding of what disease is and how Nature tries to overcome it, the veterinarian directs his efforts at assisting Nature. He tries to find out why a heart is beating faster than it normally should, rather than just giving a drug that will slow it down. He looks for the reason when an animal has quit eating, instead of prescribing some medicine that is said to stimulate the appetite. What was once mainly an art has become a science and an art.

DRUGS that act on or affect organs or tissues with which they come in direct contact at the time they are used are said to exert local action.

Drugs that are absorbed into the blood stream and are distributed throughout the body before results are produced are said to be systemic or general in their effects.

Drugs and medicines may be classified according to the actions they produce in the treated animal. Many of the terms used to describe such actions are well known. Stimulant, depressant, anesthetic, blister, irritant, antiseptic, narcotic, and antibiotic need little explanation.

Probably most of the drugs used in treating domestic animals are stimulants. Examples are laxatives or purgatives, which stimulate the bowels; diuretics, which stimulate the kidneys; diaphoretics, which stimulate sweating; and expectorants, which stimulate glandular secretion.

Many drugs have more than a single action. Turpentine is a fairly effective treatment for the coughing that accompanies certain types of laryngitis or pharyngitis, but it is an irritant to the kidneys. Alcohol is a depressant if given internally, but it is a mild local stimulant when it is applied to the skin. Some of the most active of the antibiotics have harmful side reactions, so that they must be used with a great deal of caution.

A few drugs are used as direct replacements for necessary constituents of the normal body. The treatment that is perhaps the most dramatic one in the whole field of medicine the intravenous injection of some form of soluble calcium in a cow with parturient paresis (milk fever) is in this group. As soon as the calcium content of the circulating blood is raised significantly, the cow that is being treated usually shows some response. It is not unusual for an animal that appeared on the verge of death and that probably would have died within a few hours if left untreated to be on her feet in 10 to 15 minutes after the injection is completed. Many of the hormones are in this group, too. Spectacular effects follow the administration of thyroxin, the secretion of the thyroid gland, to animals suffering from thyroid deficiency.

Administration of drugs to farm animals often is a rather serious problem. Theoretically drugs can be given to livestock by any and all the routes that they can be given to human patients, such as by the mouth, by injection with a hypodermic syringe, by inhalation, or by direct application. But there are many reasons why the veterinarian cannot leave drugs for owners to give to their animals by mouth just as the physician leaves medicine for his human patients to take that way.

Perhaps the best way for the average owner to give medicine to his livestock or poultry by mouth is to mix it with feed or salt or give it in the drinking water. But this can be done only in cases in which the animal is taking feed, licking salt, or drinking. It is not very useful in the acutely and seriously sick, which neither eat nor drink. Nor can drugs which have such disagreeable flavours or odours that animals refuse to take them be given in this manner. Sometimes flavours can be disguised by mixing a little blackstrap molasses with the feed, water, or salt. The use of salt as a vehicle for giving such needed elements as iron, copper, cobalt, and iodine now is standard practice. Some worm remedies, particularly phenothiazine, are taken rather readily by sheep and somewhat less so by cattle when they are mixed with salt.

None of the farm animals, except dogs, will take bad-tasting drugs by mouth willingly. They must be given liquids as drenches, with a dose syringe, or by a direct injection into the stomach through a stomach tube. Pills, capsules, and boluses must be placed far back in the mouth if they are to be swallowed.

All of these procedures are time consuming even to a veterinarian who is trained in ways to give medicine.

Staveley Farms Boer Goats

Lice

Symptoms: Rough coat, itching, if the animal has horns you can see little fur holes where they are scratching themselves, thin. usually more common in the fall and winter months.

Treatment: We use delice pour-on, put it in a squeeze bottle and go along all their backs careful not to put too much on. Sometimes some of them have a reaction to the treatment and loose some of their fur. But it always grows back.

Chorioptic Mange: Mites that live on the skin. Not all animals seam to get it even though they are in the same pen together. Generally is contracted in the colder weather and can live up to ten weeks.

Symptoms: Usually you see hair loss, pink irritated skin, yellow scabs on the lower legs, can be on the scrotum or utter. Treatment: Ivomec injectable give it to all animals that are in contact. It may need to re-treat in two weeks. I give each animal a dose and a half.

Pneumonia

Symptoms: Not eating, depressed, Laboured breathing, animal standing by itself, rattle in the chest, sometime coughing, sometimes nasal discharge usually fever but not always. I put my ear to the animals chest and usually I can hear if it is in the throat or in the lungs. If it's in the throat it is most likely just a common cold. They sometimes get this when the weather changes quickly or it is very wet and rainy.

The way I can usually tell the difference between if it is just a cold or pneumonia is that a normal breathing goat you can barely see the goat breathing. Look at the rest of the animals in the pen and compare how they inhale and exhale to the one in question. You should be able to see a difference between them if the goat has pneumonia.

Prevention : Well ventilated and draft free barn, dry clean bedding and no crowding. Keep all new animals coming in to your barn separate. Treatment: We use Excenel RTU it works fast and has a low withdrawl period on meat and can be stored on the shelf for a long time. It is expensive but very effective. The thing with pneumonia you don't have time to wait it comes on very quickly. Depending on the size of the animal usually a dose of around 1cc per 25 to 30lbs of goat is what I give.... So a mature doe would be treated with around 5cc and a kid 1 or 2cc per treatment. The first day or two depending on how the goat responds I give a dose AM and PM. Then once a day for usually 3 to 5 days. I have also given goats children's cold medicine to help with the congestion. The same dosage I would give a child by estimated weight.

Coccidiosis

Symptoms: Usually seen in very young kids just starting to eat feeds, but can happen to older animals as well not as common they generally develop an immunity to it. Diarrhea with blood and/or mucus, not eating well, bloaty belly poor looking coat. (these symptoms can be very similar for worm infestation as well) If they get hit with coccidiosis or a heavy worm load and are not treated quickly enough they never do well afterwards the damage is done.

Prevention : We feed our mothers Rumensin one month before kidding to lower the load in the pens. Keep feeders and waters clean and pens dry don't over crowd. The reality of it is once you have goats for a few years you will have coccidiosis all farms do no matter how clean your facilities are it is like worms. It is a matter of knowing how to manage and treat for it.

Treatment: We have a medicated feed for our kids that has Rumensin added as a preventative but sometimes they don't eat enough creep when they are small to prevent it just the same so we treat them by mouth with Sulfa drugs. Sulfa 25% solution administer 45 ml per 100lbs (about 10cc per 20 25lb kid) first day then 1/2 the dose for no more than 5 days, most of the time you only need one or two treatments.

We also give Dairymans Choice vitamin and enzyme supplement for cattle at the same time 5grms so that they are not lacking. We use to use Decox powder given directly in the mouth usually 1/2 teaspoon per day per kid but found it took longer to work. Sometime we give electrolytes as well.

E.Coli: Looks very similar to Coccidiosis but the diarrhea has a very strong odour and is yellow coloured. Treat with decox and electrolytes sometimes antibiotics is needed as well.

Worms

Symptoms: Thinner than rest of herd for no reason, white eyes should have pink or red under bottom eye lid, coughing, anemia pale pink or grey gums, bottle jaw swelling under chin at night means it is filling up with fluid, not eating, rough coat, diarrhea.

Prevention : Keep an eye on your stock don't wait to treat if an animal looks a bit thinner for no reason. Check the eyes and the gums. I found treating one or two animals that need it rather than treating all of them works best that way their is less resistance built up against the de-wormers. We rotate our pastures so that the grass never gets to low, that way they are not eating as much worm larva.

Treatment: We use Cydectin and treat as needed. Not all animals. Give a dose and a half to the ones that need it. For young kids usually we weigh them regularly and if there is one that is not growing as well it gets treated.

Navel III

Symptoms: Swelling and pain in one or more joints in young kids. It is usually the cause of infection in the umbilical cord from early on at birth or soon afterwards. Sometimes it is months later before they have symptoms of sore legs and swelling.

Prevention : Dip navel cords in iodine when the kids are first born. Keep birthing pens clean and dry even doing this they can still get it but less likely.

Treatment: Give injections of antibiotics for one to two weeks, prognoses is not good.

Clouded eyes : I have had kids born with clouded eyes, I'm not sure what the actual name for this condition is but we use "Special Formula" it is an antibiotic cow utter treatment for mastitis. Just put it right in the eye twice a day for several days. It clears it up in no time.

Urinary Calculi

Symptoms: young male or withered goats stretch out trying to urinate but very little is coming out, bloody urine, not eating, in pain swollen underneath because of urinary stones that are causing blockage. Over time the animal stops eating and drinking and urine builds up behind the stone causing either the bladder or urethra to rupture.

Prevention : Make sure there is always fresh water and minerals, be careful not to have an imbalance of feed the total ration should have a 2:1 or 2:5:1 calcium: phosphorus ration. The animals should always have a good amount of hay to eat ,to much grain is usually the cause of this to young bucks. Salt added to the feed makes them drink more so they are less likely to have a blockage, ammonia Chloride can be added to your feed if you have a reoccurring problem with this.

Treatment

Not usually good news... If it is in the urethral process and it is not a hard stone it maybe possible to gently squeeze it out or the urethral process can be snipped off with a pair of scissors. The animal should be able to urinate right away. If in the case that the animal is still able to urinate, feed can be taken away for a day and it can be dosed with ammonia chloride. Otherwise their are surgical procedures that your vet can do but in most cases the outcome is not good.

Listeriosis: (Circling Disease)

Symptoms: Depression, disorientation, stargazing, staggering, weaving, circling, one sided facial paralysis. Prevention :Be very careful not to feed moldy hay or feed of any kind usually it is from silage, sometimes it doesn't take much just a bit. Don't make drastic changes in the type or amount of feed. Treatment: Antiobotics: Tetracycline or penicillin Large dose every six hours first three to five days then daily for seven days.

Mastitis

Symptoms: Swollen red hot utter, fever, clumps or blood in the milk, doe off her feed and depressed. Prevention: Cut the feed ration down by at least 1/2 at weaning time switch from legume hay to grass. Some times if it's feasible leave one kid on for a week longer so that the doe has a chance to slow down her milk production. We have culled does out for having large or any problem utters that don't dry up after the kids are weaned. It can be just to much trouble.

Treatment: When we first started in goats we had a bunch of old dairy animals with huge utters that drug almost on the ground. I learned that mastitis can be caused by Staph, Strept or E-coli and the type of antibiotics is different depending on which kind it is. My first choice was usually Penicillin G twice a day large doses of 5 or 6cc as well as intramammary infusion tubes. If this doesn't work in a few days then you have to try another type of injectable antibiotic. But in my experience if you wait to treat while you do a culture on the bacteria your doe is going to be very sick and maybe die anyways. Milk out the utter twice a day into a container to remove the infection, careful dispose of it don't milk it on the ground you don't want to contaminate the pen. Continue to insert the infusion tubes twice a day for several days each time you milk the doe out.

If it is gangrenous mastitis you need to treat it very aggressively with antibiotics call your vet. The skin over the infected half will turn blue and cold and if the goat survives most of the time the affected tissue will no longer be functional. Sometimes the tissue affected on one side will be so badly damaged that it will die and fall off and the doe will still live.

Colic

Symptoms: The problem is that the goat is full of gas and can't get it to come out of it's largest stomach. It has a swollen bloated belly, grinding teeth, stretching out it's body and straining trying to go but nothing comes out, not eating, kicking at it's sides, laying down and moaning in pain.

Prevention: Give goats dry hay before going out onto lush pasture so that they are less likely to gorge. Never give too much grain or change ration too quickly. Goats are very sensitive to feed changes.

Treatment: I usually treat goats with 1/2 cup of mineral oil and 2 table spoons of baking soda. You can also use pepto bismol 1 to 2 teaspoons. Rub the belly and try and keep the animal moving by walking it around. Stand the animal on a hill facing upwards it will help to get it to burp. This method takes time so be patient it usually work with in a few hours the goat is eating hay again.

Tubing is also possible but I have never had to do this and it is best if some one that has experience show you how or call your vet. This is a very serious illness don't wait to treat your animal or they will most likely die.

What is Anthrax?

Anthrax is a life-threatening infectious disease that normally affects animals, especially ruminants (such as goats, cattle, sheep, and horses). Anthrax can be transmitted to humans by contact with infected animals or their products. In recent years, anthrax has received a great deal of attention as it has become clear that the infection can also be spread by a bioterrorist attack or by biological warfare. Anthrax does not spread from person to person.

What Causes Anthrax?

The agent of anthrax is a bacterium called *Bacillus anthracis.* While other investigators discovered the anthrax bacillus, it was a German physician and scientist, Dr. Robert Koch, who proved that the anthrax bacterium was the cause of a disease that affected farm animals in his community. Under the microscope, the bacteria look like large rods. However, in the soil, where they live, anthrax organisms exist in a dormant form called spores. These spores are very hardy and difficult to destroy. The spores have been known to survive in the soil for as long as 48 years.

How is Anthrax Contracted?

Anthrax can infect humans in three ways. The most common is infection through the skin, which causes an ugly sore that usually goes away without treatment. Humans and animals can ingest anthrax from carcasses of dead animals that have been contaminated with anthrax. Ingestion of anthrax can cause serious, sometimes fatal disease. The most deadly form is inhalation anthrax. If the spores of anthrax are inhaled, they migrate to lymph glands in the chest where they proliferate, spread, and produce toxins that often cause death.

How Common is Anthrax?

Anthrax is now rare in humans in the United States and developed countries. It still occurs today, largely in countries lacking public-health regulations that prevent exposure to infected goats, cattle, sheep, and horses and their products. In the last few years, there have been rare cases of anthrax in people exposed to imported animal hides used to make drums. Drum players, drum makers, and their family members have been infected in this way. The major concern for those of us in western countries (who don't play drums) is the use of anthrax as an agent of biological warfare.

How Long is the Incubation Period with Anthrax?

The incubation period (the period between contact with anthrax and the start of symptoms) may be relatively short, from one to five days. Like other infectious diseases, the incubation period for anthrax is quite variable and it may be weeks before an infected individual feels sick.

What Kinds of Diseases does Anthrax Cause?

There are three forms of disease caused by anthrax: cutaneous (skin) anthrax, inhalation anthrax, and gastrointestinal (bowel) anthrax.

Cutaneous Anthrax

The cutaneous (skin) form of anthrax starts as a red-brown raised spot that enlarges with considerable redness around it, blistering, and hardening. The centre of the spot then shows an ulcer crater with blood-tinged drainage and the formation of a black crust called an eschar. There are swollen glands (lymph nodes) in the area. Symptoms include muscle aches and pain, headache, fever, nausea, and vomiting. The illness usually resolves in about six weeks, but deaths may occur if patients do not receive appropriate antibiotics.

Inhalation Anthrax

The first symptoms are subtle, gradual and flu-like (influenza). In a few days, however, the illness worsens and there may be severe respiratory distress. Shock, coma, and death follow. Inhalation anthrax does not cause a true pneumonia. In fact, the spores get picked in the lungs up by scavenger cells called macrophages. Most of the spores are killed. Unfortunately, some survive and are transported to glands in the chest called lymph nodes. In the lymph nodes, the spores that survive multiply, produce deadly toxins, and spread throughout the body. Severe hemorrhage and tissue death (necrosis) occurs in these lymph nodes in the chest. From there, the disease spreads to the adjacent lungs and the rest of the body. Inhalation anthrax is a very serious disease, and unfortunately, most affected individuals will die even if they get appropriate antibiotics. Why is this so? The antibiotics are effective in killing the bacteria, but they do not destroy the deadly toxins that have already been released by the anthrax bacteria.

Gastrointestinal Anthrax

Now rare, anthrax of the bowels (gastrointestinal anthrax) is the result of eating undercooked, contaminated meat. The symptoms of this form of anthrax include nausea, loss of appetite, bloody diarrhea and fever followed by abdominal pain. The bacteria invade through the bowel wall. Then the infection spreads throughout the body through the bloodstream (septicemia) with deadly toxicity.

How is the Diagnosis Made of Anthrax?

The history, including the occupation of the person, is important. The bacteria may be found in cultures or smears in cutaneous (skin) anthrax and in throat swabs and sputum in pulmonary anthrax. Chest X-rays may also show characteristic changes in and between the lungs. Once the anthrax is disseminated, bacteria can be seen in the blood using a microscope. Of course, if anthrax is deliberately spread, the manifestations of the disease may be unusual. Indeed, in the bioterrorism attack in the U.S. in 2001, anthrax spores were spread through the postal system as a white powder mailed with letters.

How is Anthrax Treated?

In most cases, early treatment can cure anthrax. The cutaneous (skin) form of anthrax can be treated with common antibiotics such as penicillin, tetracycline, erythromycin, and ciprofloxacin (Cipro). The pulmonary form of anthrax is a medical emergency. Early and continuous intravenous therapy with antibiotics may be lifesaving. In a bioterrorism attack, individuals exposed to anthrax will be given antibiotics before they become sick. A vaccine exists but is not yet available to the general public. Most experts think that the vaccine will also be given to exposed individuals who are victims of a bioterrorist attack. Of note, anthrax is a reportable disease. That means that local or state health agencies must be notified if a case of anthrax is diagnosed. These agencies can better characterise the anthrax so that the affected individual can receive the most effective treatment for that particular organism.

How can Anthrax be Prevented?

Public-health measures to prevent contact with infected animals are invaluable. There is a vaccine available for people at high risk (such as veterinarians, laboratory technicians, employees of textile mills processing imported goat hair, and members of the armed forces). The Department of Defence and the U.S. Centres for Disease Control and Prevention are working very hard to prevent a bioterrorist attack and to be prepared to deal with the consequences if one occurs.

For anthrax and other infectious diseases, vaccines with greater efficacy and fewer side effects are under development. Currently, most vaccines are given by injection into fat or muscle below the skin. Early studies in experimental animals are showing promise for an oral vaccine for anthrax. Obviously, a pill is easier to take than a shot, and the pill may even be a safer and more effective route of administration.

Anthrax at a Glance

- Anthrax is an infection by bacteria transmitted from animals.
- Anthrax causes skin, lung, and bowel disease and can be deadly.
- Anthrax is diagnosed by cultures from infected tissues.
- Anthrax is treated by antibiotics.
- Anthrax can be prevented.
- Sadly, the greatest threat of anthrax today is through a bioterrorist attack.
- Federal, state, and local agencies are working hard to deal with this bioterrorist threat.

What are the Treatments for MS Disease?

MS, or multiple sclerosis, is a disease that causes the immune system to eat away at the sheath that protects the nerves. This disease ultimately can cause the nerves to deteriorate.

Cause

According to the Mayo Clinic, the exact cause for MS is unknown. Genetics and infections are believed to play a role. Other factors that contribute to the development of MS might include thyroid disease, inflammatory bowel disease and type 1 diabetes.

Treatment

There are many treatment options available for MS, though there is no cure. These treatment options include numerous types of medication, therapy and surgical procedures.

Function

The medications prescribed for MS work by relieving the symptoms of MS, such as pain, fatigue, dizziness, weakness and tremors, and by helping slow down the disease. Therapy includes strengthening and stretching the muscles to help in the performance of daily activities. Plasma exchange, a procedure that separates the plasma from the blood, might help fight the symptoms of MS relapses.

Side Effects

Many of these medications can cause negative effects such as liver damage, shortness of breath, flushing or leukoencephalopathy, a brain infection that can be fatal.

What are the Treatments for Cushing's Disease?

Cushing's Disease is a glandular problem. When pituitary or adrenal glands malfunction, they can secrete too many hormones. These hormones affect a dog's metabolism and health and can cause hyperadrenocorticism, commonly called Cushing's Disease. Without treatment Cushing's can spur more complicated diseases like diabetes, kidney failure and heart disease.

Symptoms

Typically, the dog owner sees hair loss and behavioural changes in the dog. The dog is eagerly hungry and thirsty. He drinks water constantly and urinates often. He is overstimulated by excess hormones and may be hyperactive. Over a period of weeks the dog develops a potbelly and muscles waste away. Meanwhile, his hair falls out or becomes brittle.

Diagnosis

When the owner takes the dog to a vet, the disease may not be easily diagnosed. Diabetes and other diseases have similar symptoms to Cushing's. The veterinarian will need to do several tests to find the specific disease troubling the dog, including a urinalysis, blood chemistry panel and other clinical tests measuring gland activity.

When Cushing's disease is confirmed, the veterinarian determines whether steroid drugs, pituitary gland tumours or adrenal tumours caused the disease. The treatment for Cushing's depends on the cause.

Iatrogenic Treatment

The easiest type of Cushing's to treat is caused by steroid or corticosteroid drugs such as prednisone. These drugs cause iatrogenic Cushing's by overstimulating the glands. Lowering the drug dose or giving it less often until the glands return to normal levels controls Cushing's.

Pituitary Treatment

The most common type of Cushing's is caused by benign tumours on the pituitary gland. The gland puts out too much cortisone. Drugs usually treat this type of Cushing's. The traditional drug is Lysodren, but newer drugs include Trilostane, Ketoconazole and Anipryl. Each drug has pros and cons.

The veterinarian may run a series of tests to find the drug and dosage suited to the dog—and to the owner's lifestyle. These medications are often costly and require precise dosage that not everyone can manage.

Less-common treatments include radiation or holistic herbs. Radiation is costly and must be repeated under anesthesia, often hazardous for older dogs that commonly develop Cushing's. Herbal medications have strong effects on the dog and can, like prescription drugs, be lethal if not properly monitored.

Adrenal Treatment

Adrenal tumours, less common than pituitary tumours, are sometimes removed by surgery. In about half of cases with adrenal tumours, the tumour is malignant and cancer may be in vital organs. Surgery does not offer much benefit for these dogs and is an added stress to the dog and his owner. Short-term medication may be suggested by the veterinarian depending on canine pain or discomfort.

Considerations

Treating Cushing's Disease is challenging, time-consuming and costly. In many cases proper treatment significantly improves the dog's quality of life and adds years to his lifespan. In some cases, an older dog has other serious problems. The owner may decide not to treat Cushing's Disease; the dog may eventually die of more serious complications or may need to be euthanized.

What are the Treatments for Kawasaki Disease ?

Kawasaki disease, which includes blood vessel inflammation, is a lymph node syndrome that most commonly occurs in children. Some of the symptoms involve high fever, bloodshot eyes, changes in the lips, coating on the tongue, swollen lymph nodes and peeling skin. For some patients with Kawasaki disease, complications can include inflammation of the heart lining, joint inflammation and meningitis.

Treatment

Diagnosis and treatment of Kawasaki disease is especially important in the first 10 days of symptoms. Treatment is vital to avoid damage to the cardiovascular system, which often involves heart damage and changes in the blood vessels. Sufferers are often admitted to the hospital for treatment once a diagnosis has been made.

Medication

High doses of an IV of gamma globulin is one of the standard treatments. This lowers the risk of coronary artery problems and decreases blood vessel inflammation. This treatment necessitates a one-day stay in the hospital if the patient's condition improves. Gamma globulin is most effective if given before the tenth day of fever. If the fever does not dissipate, another round may be required.

Aspirin is often given as part of the treatment to help prevent blood clots and decrease pain, fever and inflammation. If no complications exist, the dosages are reduced and are taken for two to three months.

Anticoagulants can help reduce the risk of an aneurysm and prevent the formation of new blood clots.

Plasmapheresis

Plasma exchange, also called plasmapheresis, is a treatment option made available for patients who have been unresponsive to gamma globulin, aspirin and anticoagulant medication. This process removes plasma from the blood and replaces it with protein. During plasmapheresis, antibodies and proteins in the blood can also be removed.

TNF Blocking Drugs

This medication blocks the effects of a molecule that acts as a messenger of inflammation. TNF blocking medication is being reviewed for its effectiveness and is not yet part of the treatment process (as of 2009).

Follow-Up

Echocardiograms are a regular part of follow-up treatment plans to check for aneurysms. This is normally done up to eight weeks after the onset of Kawasaki disease.

Acute Kawasaki disease often requires several years of follow-up and care, depending on what affect the disease had on the body. Medicine, limitations on physical activity and ongoing tests may be required. However, most patients with Kawasaki disease are able to return to normal activity.

Considerations

The IV of gamma globulin can interfere with immunisation effectiveness and may lower the patient's level of immunity. Immunisations should be halted for 11 months after the treatment of the acute phase.

Actinomycetes

Nocardiosis is commonly reported in debilitated marine mammals. It has been diagnosed in bottlenose dolphins, beluga whales, pilot whales (Globicephala spp), harbor porpoises, killer whales (Orcinus orca), false killer whales (Pseudorca crassidens), spinner dolphins (Stenella longirostris), and leopard seals (Hydrurga leptonyx). Infections due to Actinomyces spp also have been diagnosed in bottlenose dolphins.

Brucellosis

Brucellosis is a relatively recent development in marine mammals, with initial reports of serologic evidence of the disease in 1994. Since that time, a wide range of pinniped and cetacean species have been shown to have antibodies to Brucella spp . Several marine Brucella species have been cultured, and genetic analyses show these to be different from known terrestrial Brucella spp . Strains from dolphins, porpoises, and pinnipeds appear to be distinct from each other, but strains from one type of animal do not seem to vary much from the Atlantic to the Pacific ocean.

Diagnosis remains controversial with challenges in both culture techniques and serologic methods. Little is known about the pathophysiology of brucellosis in marine mammals, although some postulate that transitory reproductive dysfunction is a component of the disease. Clinical experience with the disease is not extensive and no therapy or control methods are established. Zoonotic potential has not yet been determined.

Clostridial Myositis

Severe myositis due to infections with Clostridium spp has been diagnosed in captive killer whales, pilot whales, bottlenose dolphins, California sea lions, and manatees. All marine mammals are probably susceptible. The disease is characterised by acute swelling, muscle necrosis, and accumulations of gas in affected tissues, accompanied by a severe leukocytosis. Untreated, it can be fatal. Diagnosis is based on detection of gram-positive bacilli in aspirates of the lesions and is confirmed by anaerobic culture and identification of the organism. Treatment includes systemic and local antibiotics, surgical drainage of abscessed areas, and flushing with hydrogen peroxide. Commercially available, inactivated clostridial bacterins are used routinely in some facilities, although efficacy in

Pneumonia

The chief cause of death in captive marine mammals is believed to be pneumonia. It is not common in polar bears. Most cases of marine mammal pneumonia have significant bacterial involvement, and most organisms cultured from terrestrial species have been identified in marine mammals. Pneumonia often can be considered the result of mismanagement. Marine mammals require good air quality, including high rates of air exchange at the water surface in indoor facilities. Tempered air or acclimation to cold temperatures is also important to prevent lung disease, even in polar species.

Animals acclimated to cold temperatures are usually quite hardy; however, sudden transition from warm environments to cold air, even with warmer water, can precipitate fulminating pneumonias, particularly in nutritionally or otherwise compromised animals. Clinical signs include lethargy, anorexia, severe halitosis, dyspnea, pyrexia, and marked leukocytosis. The disease can progress rapidly. Diagnosis is usually based on clinical signs and confirmed by response to therapy. Treatment consists of correction of environmental factors and intensive antibiotic and supportive therapy. The initial antibiotic is usually broad-spectrum, commonly cephalexin (40 mg/kg, tid or qid); adjustments are based on cultures and sensitivities from blowhole or tracheal samples.

Erysipelas (Diamond Skin Disease)

Erysipelas can be a serious infectious disease of captive cetaceans and pinnipeds. The organism, Erysipelothrix rhusiopathiae , which causes erysipelas in pigs and other domestic species, is a common contaminant of fish. A septicemic form of the disease in marine mammals can be peracute or acute; affected animals die suddenly either with no prodromal signs or with sudden depression, inappetence, or fever. A cutancous form that causes typical rhomboidal skin lesions is a more chronic form of the disease. Animals with this form usually recover with timely antibiotic treatment.

Necropsy of peracute cases generally fails to reveal grossly discernible lesions other than widespread petechiation. Diagnosis is based on culture of the organism from the blood, spleen, or body cavities. Arthritis has been found in animals that have died with the chronic form. Treatment of the peracute and acute forms has rarely been attempted because the absence of prodromal signs obscures the diagnosis. Animals with the dermatologic form usually recover with administration of penicillins, tetracyclines, or chloramphenicol and supportive treatment.

Leptospirosis

This has been diagnosed in otarid pinnipeds and bears. In seals, the disease is characterised by depression, reluctance to move, polydipsia, and pyrexia. It may also cause abortions and neonatal deaths in California sea lions and Northern fur seals. Lesions include a severe, diffuse, interstitial nephritis, with renal tubules packed with spirochetes.

The gallbladder may contain inspissated black bile, but hepatitis may not be apparent grossly. Hyperplasia of Kupffer's cells, erythrophagocytosis, and hemosiderosis are seen histologically. Gastroenteritis can be a feature. Antibodies to various Leptospira serovars (L canicola , L icterohaemorrhagiae , L autumnalis , and L pomona) have been identified in affected animals by fluorescent antibody techniques. Treatment in pinnipeds is similar to that in dogs Control in captive animals

Streptothricosis (Dolphin Pseudopox, Cutaneous Dermatophilosis)

Streptothricosis (Dermatophilus congolensis), a subcutaneous bacterial disease, has been reported in pinnipeds and polar bears. It must be distinguished from sealpox. Simultaneous infections of streptothricosis and pox have been recorded in sea lions. Cutaneous streptothricosis usually manifests as sharply delineated nodules distributed over the entire body and usually progresses to death. Diagnosis is based on demonstration of the organism in biopsies or culture. Treatment with prolonged high dosages of systemic antibiotics can be successful. Sporothrix schenckii , the cause of a subcutaneous mycosis, has been reported in Pacific white-sided dolphins (Laegenorhynchus obliquidens).

Tuberculosis

Marine mammals are susceptible to various mycobacteria. Unconfirmed tuberculosis has been reported in a stranded, wild bottlenose dolphin in the Mediterranean, and indirect evidence points to Mycobacterium tuberculosis being possibly endemic in free-ranging otarids off the coast of Australia. (Originally thought to be M bovis , subsequent molecular assessment places the isolates from free-ranging southern hemisphere pinnipeds in a unique cluster in the M tuberculosis complex.)

Subantarctic fur seals (Arctocephalus tropicalis)) are thought to be the common link in the spread of the disease to other pinniped species because they cohabit with the other known affected species, Australian sean lions (Neophoca cinerea) and New Zealand fur seals (Arctocephalus forsteri). Otherwise, mycobacteriosis has been a disease of captivity. Pinnipeds, cetaceans, and sirenians have developed disease due to M bovis , M smegmatis ,

There are strong indications that immunosuppression may be involved in the development of infections by the atypical mycobacteria. Intradermal testing with high concentrations of bovine or avian purified protein derivative tuberculin can be used to screen exposed animals; however, anergy occurs. In pinnipeds, injections in the webbing of the rear flippers should be read at 48 and 72 hr. ELISA screening has identified antibodies in seals but requires further evaluation before it can be considered a screening test. Diagnosis is made by culture and identification of the organism from lesion biopsies, tracheal washes, or feces. Mycobacteriosis in marine mammals is an emerging disease and is probably of public health significance

Miscellaneous Bacterial Diseases

Marine mammals are probably susceptible to the entire range of pathogenic bacteria. Pasteurella multocida has caused several outbreaks of hemorrhagic enteritis with depression and abdominal distress leading to acute death in dolphins and pinnipeds. It has also been reported to cause pneumonia in pinnipeds. In dolphins, Mannheimia (Pasteurella) haemolytica has been incriminated in hemorrhagic tracheitis that responded to chloramphenicol therapy

Chapter 5

Diseases from Farm Animals

Farm animals including cows, sheep, pigs, chickens and goats, can pass diseases to people. As you know, farm animals are not like house pets and do not have places to rest or eat that are away from where they pass manure. Therefore, you should thoroughly wash your hands with running water and soap after contact with them or after touching things such as fences, buckets, and straw bedding, that have been in contact with farm animals, adults should carefully watch children who are visiting farms and help them wash their hands well.

Different types of farm animals can carry different diseases. For example, cows and calves can carry the bacterium *Escherichia coli* O157:H7, often called *E. coli* (ee COH-lie). This germ can cause bloody diarrhea in people. In addition children can develop kidney failure due to *E. coli* O157:H7 infection. Pigs can carry the bacterium *Yersinia enterocolitica* (yer-SIN-ee-ah en-TER-o-koh-LIH-tee-kuh), which causes the disease yersiniosis (yer-SIN-ee-OH-sis). Chickens can carry bacteria such as Salmonella, (sal –mon – Nell – ah) which causes the disease salmonellosis. Many of these germs are in farm animal manure.

Some people are more likely than others to get diseases from farm animals. A person's age and health status may affect his or her immune system, increasing the chances of getting sick. People who are more likely to get diseases from farm animals include infants, children younger than 5 years old, organ transplant patients, people with HIV/AIDS, and people who are being treated for cancer. Special advice is available for people who are at greater risk than others of getting diseases from animals.

BSE (Bovine Spongiform Encephalopathy, or Mad Cow Disease)

BSE (bovine spongiform encephalopathy) is a progressive neurological disorder of cattle that results from infection by an unusual transmissible agent called a prion. The nature of the transmissible agent is not well understood. Currently, the most accepted theory is that the agent is a modified form of a normal protein known as prion protein. For reasons that are not yet understood, the normal prion protein changes into a pathogenic (harmful) form that then damages the central nervous system of cattle.

Research indicates that the first probable infections of BSE in cows occurred during the 1970's with two cases of BSE being identified in 1986. BSE possibly originated as a result of feeding cattle meat-and-bone meal that contained BSE-infected products from a spontaneously occurring case of BSE or scrapie-infected sheep products. Scrapie is a prion disease of sheep. There is strong evidence and general agreement that the outbreak was then amplified and spread throughout the United Kingdom cattle industry by feeding rendered, prion-infected, bovine meat-and-bone meal to young calves.

The BSE epizootic in the United Kingdom peaked in January 1993 at almost 1,000 new cases per week. Over the next 17 years, the annual numbers of BSE cases has dropped sharply; 14,562 cases in 1995, 1,443 in 2000, 225 in 2005 and 11 cases in 2010. Cumulatively, through the end of 2010, more than 184,500 cases of BSE had been confirmed in the United Kingdom alone in more than 35,000 herds.

There exists strong epidemiologic and laboratory evidence for a causal association between a new human prion disease called variant Creutzfeldt-Jakob disease (vCJD) that was first reported from the United Kingdom in 1996 and the BSE outbreak in cattle. The interval between the most likely period for the initial extended exposure of the population to potentially BSE-contaminated food (1984-1986) and the onset of initial variant CJD cases (1994-1996) is consistent with known incubation periods for the human forms of prion disease.

BSE (bovine spongiform encephalopathy) is a progressive neurological disorder of cattle that results from infection by an unusual transmissible agent called a prion. The nature of the transmissible agent is not well understood. Currently, the most accepted theory is that the agent is a modified form of a normal protein known as prion protein. For reasons that are not yet understood, the normal prion protein changes into a pathogenic (harmful) form that then damages the central nervous system of cattle.

Research indicates that the first probable infections of BSE in cows occurred during the 1970's with two cases of BSE being identified in 1986. BSE possibly originated as a result of feeding cattle meat-and-bone meal that contained BSE-infected products from a spontaneously occurring case of BSE or scrapie-infected sheep products. Scrapie is a prion disease of sheep. There is strong evidence and general agreement that the outbreak was then amplified and spread throughout the United Kingdom cattle industry by feeding rendered, prion-infected, bovine meat-and-bone meal to young calves.

The BSE epizootic in the United Kingdom peaked in January 1993 at almost 1,000 new cases per week. Over the next 17 years, the annual numbers of BSE cases has dropped sharply; 14,562 cases in 1995, 1,443 in 2000, 225 in 2005 and 11 cases in 2010. Cumulatively, through the end of 2010, more than 184,500 cases of BSE had been confirmed in the United Kingdom alone in more than 35,000 herds.

There exists strong epidemiologic and laboratory evidence for a causal association between a new human prion disease called variant Creutzfeldt-Jakob disease (vCJD) that was first reported from the United Kingdom in 1996 and the BSE outbreak in cattle.

The interval between the most likely period for the initial extended exposure of the population to potentially BSE-contaminated food (1984-1986) and the onset of initial variant CJD cases (1994-1996) is consistent with known incubation periods for the human forms of prion disease.

BSE (bovine spongiform encephalopathy) is a progressive neurological disorder of cattle that results from infection by an unusual transmissible agent called a prion. The nature of the transmissible agent is not well understood. Currently, the most accepted theory is that the agent is a modified form of a normal protein known as prion protein. For reasons that are not yet understood, the normal prion protein changes into a pathogenic (harmful) form that then damages the central nervous system of cattle.

Research indicates that the first probable infections of BSE in cows occurred during the 1970's with two cases of BSE being identified in 1986. BSE possibly originated as a result of feeding cattle meat-and-bone meal that contained BSE-infected products from a spontaneously occurring case of BSE or scrapie-infected sheep products. Scrapie is a prion disease of sheep. There is strong evidence and general agreement that the outbreak was then amplified and spread throughout the United Kingdom cattle industry by feeding rendered, prion-infected, bovine meat-and-bone meal to young calves.

The BSE epizootic in the United Kingdom peaked in January 1993 at almost 1,000 new cases per week. Over the next 17 years, the annual numbers of BSE cases has dropped sharply; 14,562 cases in 1995, 1,443 in 2000, 225 in 2005 and 11 cases in 2010. Cumulatively, through the end of 2010, more than 184,500 cases of BSE had been confirmed in the United Kingdom alone in more than 35,000 herds.

There exists strong epidemiologic and laboratory evidence for a causal association between a new human prion disease called variant Creutzfeldt-Jakob disease (vCJD) that was first reported from the United Kingdom in 1996 and the BSE outbreak in cattle. The interval between the most likely period for the initial extended exposure of the population to potentially BSE-contaminated food (1984-1986) and the onset of initial variant CJD cases (1994-1996) is consistent with known incubation periods for the human forms of prion disease.

Brucellosis

Clinical Features In the acute form (<8 weeks from illness onset), nonspecific and "flu-like" symptoms including fever, sweats, malaise, anorexia, headache, myalgia, and back pain. In the undulant form (<1 year from illness onset), symptoms include undulant fevers, arthritis, and epididymo-orchitis in males. Neurologic symptoms may occur acutely in up to 5% of cases.

In the chronic form (>1 year from onset), symptoms may include chronic fatigue syndrome, depression, and arthritis. Etiologic Agent *Brucella* species, usually *B. abortus* (cattle), *B. melitensis, B.ovis* (sheep, and goats), *B. suis* (pigs), and rarely *B. canis* (dogs). Incidence In the United States, < 0.5 cases per 100,000 population, primarily *B. melitensis*. . Most cases are reported from California, Florida, Texas, and Virginia. Sequelae Variable, including granulomatous hepatitis, peripheral arthritis, spondylitis, anemia, leukopenia, thrombocytopenia, meningitis, uveitis, optic neuritis, papilledema, and endocarditis.

Transmission Zoonotic. Commonly transmitted through abrasions of the skin from handling infected mammals. In the United States, occurs more frequently by ingesting unpasteurised milk or dairy products. Highly infectious in the laboratory via aerosolisation; handling cultures warrants biosafety level-3 precautions. Risk Groups Abattoir workers, meat inspectors, animal handlers, veterinarians, and laboratorians. Surveillance Brucellosis is a nationally notifiable disease and reportable to the local health authority. Trends For previous 10 years, approximately 100 cases per year have been reported. Challenges Elimination of domestic and feral animal reservoirs. In 2001, the National Brucellosis Eradication Program reported only 3 newly affected cattle herds, compared to 14 herds identified in 2000. Establish and validate methods for isolation and detection of *Brucella* spp. in foods. Opportunities Validation of rapid diagnostic technologies developed for

Campylobacter Infection and Animals

Campylobacteriosis is a bacterial disease caused by *Campylobacter jejuni* or *Campylobacter coli*. *Campylobacter* usually causes a mild to severe infection of the gastrointestinal system, including watery or bloody diarrhea, fever, abdominal cramps, nausea, and vomiting. A rare complication of *Campylobacter* infection is Guillain-Barre syndrome, a nervous system disease that occurs approximately 2 weeks after the initial illness develops.

Can Animals Transmit Campylobacter to Me?

Sometimes, yes, animals can spread *Campylobacter* to humans. Most people get campylobacteriosis from contaminated food. However, animals can have *Campylobacter* in their feces (stool). If people touch contaminated feces, they can get sick. Animals that may carry *Campylobacter* in their feces include farm animals, cats, and dogs.

Animals do not have to be ill to pass *Campylobacter* to humans. People with compromised immune systems, including those undergoing treatments for cancer, organ transplant patients, and people with HIV/AIDS, have a higher risk than others of getting *Campylobacter* infection from food and animals.

Campylobacter Jujuni

How do I reduce my risk of getting *Campylobacter* infection from animals?

- After contact with animals and animal feces, wash your hands thoroughly with running water and soap.
- If you are immunocompromised and are getting a new pet, avoid farm animals, cats, and dogs with diarrhea.
- If your dog or cat has diarrhea, talk to your veterinarian.
- If you develop symptoms, including diarrhea, vomiting, abdominal cramps, and/or nausea, contact your physician. Be sure to inform him or her of your pet and if it is ill.
- If you are immunocompromised, be extra cautious around farm animals and their environment.

Cryptosporidium Infection and Animals

What is Cryptosporidium Infection?

Cryptosporidium infection (cryptosporidiosis) (krip-toe-spo-rid-ee-oh-sis) is a parasitic disease caused by *Cryptosporidium parvum*. It usually causes a mild to severe infection of the gastrointestinal system, including watery diarrhea, fever, abdominal cramps, nausea, and vomiting.

Can Animals Give Me Cryptosporidium Infection?

Yes, sometimes. Most people get *Cryptosporidium* infection from contaminated food and water. However, sometimes animals (including farm animals, cats, and dogs) carry this parasite in their feces (stool) and pass it to people. Animals do not have to be ill to pass *Cryptosporidium* to humans. People with compromised immune systems, such as those undergoing immunosuppressive treatments for cancer, organ transplant patients, and people with HIV/AIDS, are more likely than others to get *Cryptospordium* infection.

How do I reduce my risk of acquiring cryptosporidiosis from my pet?

- After contact with animals and animal feces (stool), wash your hands thoroughly with running water and soap.
- If you are immunocopromised and are getting a new pet, avoid strays, puppies, kittens and pets with diarrhea.
- If your dog or cat has diarrhea, take it to your veterinarian.
- If you develop symptoms, including diarrhea, vomiting, abdominal cramps, and/or nausea, contact your physician. Be sure to inform him or her of your pet and if it is ill.
- If you are immunocompromised, be extra cautious around farm animals and their environment.

How do I find more information on *Cryptosporidium* infection?

To learn more about this disease, refer to CDC's site on *Cryptosporidium* infection, including fact sheets, prevention tips, and other resources.

Escherichia Coli Infection and Farm Animals

What is Escherichia Coli O157 (E. coli)?

Escherichia coli O157 is a species of bacteria. The most common type of *E. coli* infection that causes illness in people is called *E. coli*

O157. Symptoms of *E. coli* O157 include watery or bloody diarrhea, fever, abdominal cramps, nausea, and vomiting. Illness may be mild or severe. Young children are more likely to have severe symptoms, including kidney failure, and die.

How is E. Coli Transmitted from Animals to People?

While most people get *E. coli* O157 from contaminated food (such as undercooked ground beef), it also can be passed in the manure (feces) of young calves and other cattle. Animals do not have to be ill to transmit *E. coli* O157 to humans.

How I Do Reduce My Risk of Getting E. Coli from Animals?

- After contact with cattle or their manure (feces), wash your hands thoroughly with running water and soap.
- Children under the age of 5 years old should be extra cautious around cattle (including those in petting zoos).
- If you develop symptoms, including diarrhea, vomiting, abdominal cramps, and/or nausea, contact your physician. Be sure to inform him or her of recent contact with farm animals.

How Do I Find More Information about E. Coli?

Please read CDC's *E. coli* fact sheet for answers to frequently asked questions, technical information, and references. In addition, refer to the articles below for information about *E. coli* infection at petting zoos and farms and in swimming pools.

Yersinia Enterocolitica and Pigs

What is Yersiniosis?

Yersiniosis (yer-SIN-ee-O-sis) is a disease caused by the bacterium *Yersinia enterocolitica*. People with yersiniosis can have different symptoms depending on how old they are. People can start to get sick 4 to 7 days after infection and can be sick for 1 to 3 weeks. Young children usually have fever, stomach pain, and diarrhea. Adults do not get sick with yersiniosis as often, but they can feel pain on their right side and may have a fever. Usually, these signs go away after about 3 weeks but sometimes pain in joints, such as knees or wrists, can start after that and last for several months.

Can Animals Transmit Yersiniosis to Me?

Yes, some animals pass *Yersinia enterocolitica* in their feces (stool) and people can get sick from contact with infected feces. Several kinds of animals can carry this disease, but usually people get sick from pigs that are sick with yersiniosis. Other animals that can carry this disease include cats, dogs, horses, cows, rodents, and rabbits. People can also get yersiniosis by eating pork that is not cooked completely or by drinking contaminated milk.

How Can I Protect Myself from Getting Yersiniosis?

- Avoid eating raw or undercooked pork.
- Consume only pasteurised milk or milk products.
- Wash hands with soap and running water before eating and preparing food, after contact with animals, and after handling raw meat.
- After handling raw chitterlings (food prepared from small intestine of pigs), clean hands and fingernails thoroughly with soap and water before touching infants or their toys, bottles, or pacifiers. Someone other than the foodhandler should care for children while chitterlings are being prepared.
- Prevent cross-contamination in the kitchen: Use separate cutting boards for meat and other foods, and carefully clean all cutting boards, countertops, and utensils with soap and hot water after preparing raw meat.
- Dispose of animal feces in a sanitary manner.

Infectious Cattle Diseases and Vaccines

Vaccines are available for 20 to 30 infectious diseases of cattle. With the various brand names and different combinations available, the choice of vaccines can become very complicated. Calves vaccinated under 6 months of age should generally be re-vaccinated again after that age to provide a longer lasting immunity. It is important to follow the specific directions provided with a vaccine. If two doses are recommended initially, don't count on very much protection until 7–14 days after the second dose has been given. The major diseases for which vaccines are available are categorised and briefly described below.

Sudden Death

Clostridial Diseases: These diseases include Blackleg, Malignant Edema, Black's Disease, Enterotoxemia and Redwater. All of these are common diseases. The organisms form spores that may survive a long time in hostile environments and yet kill cattle quickly, giving little opportunity for treatment. The vaccines produce good immunity, but most require two doses initially to really be effective. Some producers give only one Blackleg vaccination to calves and have no losses.

Because of the sporadic nature of these diseases, this lack of loss is probably due to a lack of exposure rather than a high level of immunity. With the other clostridial vaccines, the second dose is essential for stimulation of protective immunity (there is one designed as a one-dose vaccine).

Anthrax: This cause of sudden death has occurred in at least three areas in Utah, but is only seen sporadically. The organism will survive indefinitely in the soil and when conditions are right, multiply and cause a disease outbreak. A vaccine is available, but should only be used when cattle are grazed in known problem areas.

Respiratory Diseases

IBR (Infectious Bovine Rhinotracheitis) (Rednose): A viral infection of the upper respiratory tract. It is present in almost all herds, but causes illness in unexposed animals or those with lowered levels of immunity. Many cattle carry the virus and shed it to others during periods of stress. This agent is commonly implicated with bacterial agents in causing shipping fever and extension.usu.edu other severe cases of pneumonia.

Both MLV (modified live virus) vaccines and killed (or attenuated) products are available. Some are designed for IM (intramuscular) use while others are given IN (intranasally). The killed and intranasal products may be used in, or around, pregnant cows but other vaccines may cause abortions. The IN vaccines will cause some antibody response within three days and may be useful even in the face of an outbreak. Two doses of a killed product must be used to confer protective immunity. All replacement animals should be vaccinated. For intensively managed herds, annual boosters are recommended.

PI3 (Parainfluenza-3): Another viral respiratory agent that causes a relatively mild disease by itself, but a severe problem when combined with a bacterial agent. It is included with most IBR vaccines and can be used on the same schedule.

BVD (Bovine Virus Diarrhea): A common viral agent, present in almost all herds. It may cause respiratory, digestive tract or reproductive problems. It has a profound detrimental affect on the immune system.

A number of MLV vaccines have been available. Killed vaccines are also available which stimulate a good immune response in adult animals. But, they are apparently not able to protect the fetus. Two doses are required initially. All replacement animals should be vaccinated with an MLV vaccine (perhaps even two doses), after 6 months of age and prior to breeding.

BRSV (Bovine Respiratory Syncytial Virus): A relatively recently recognised disease agent, but now identified all across the country in respiratory infections. It is mainly a problem in weaned and feedlot animals (also young dairy stock). Both MLV and killed virus vaccines are available with two initial doses required for both. Pasteurella: A bacteria carried by many normal cattle. It becomes a major cause of severe "shipping fever" pneumonia when combined with stress and a viral agent. Two species are common: P. hemolytica and P. multocida. Vaccines available in the past were poor, with use of a single dose causing more problems than if none were used. Great improvements have been made in recent years and several newer products are available, with more to come. Both one and two dose products are now available. Follow directions carefully for these products to be beneficial. They must usually be given prior to weaning in order to help hold down the occurrence of disease at this critical time.

Haemophilus Sommus: This agent is the other major bacterial agent involved in shipping fever. It also causes "brain fever" in feedlot cattle (also known as TEME: thromboembolic meningioencephalitis). The killed vaccine must be given in two doses initially and should be used prior to weaning for the greatest benefit.

Reproductive Diseases

IBR: The most common cause of abortion in cattle. All replacements should be vaccinated to protect against it. Use the proper vaccine for, or around, pregnant cows.

BVD: May cause early embryonic death, abortion or congenital defects. Vaccinate all replacement animals with a MLV vaccine (two doses preferred) to produce a planned exposure between 6 months of age and breeding.

Brucellosis (Bangs): Many states are free of this disease agent, but vaccination is still recommended (and required for sale) until the threat from other states is further reduced. All heifers 4–12 months of age should be vaccinated by an accredited veterinarian. They must also be ear tagged and tattooed. Many states will not accept animals for breeding purposes unless the tattoo can be identified.

Vibriosis (Campylobacter): A common bacterial disease, spread through breeding. It causes early embryonic death so appears as an infertility and results in a prolonged breeding and calving season as well as a reduced calf crop. Two types of vaccine are available. One is in an oil base product to prolong the absorption. Only one dose is required initially. Subsequent boosters given in the fall at pregnancy testing will extend the protection on through the next breeding season.

The other type of vaccine has an aluminium hydroxide or other adjuvant and requires two doses initially. Be sure to give both doses to obtain a protective level of immunity. The annual boosters for this type of vaccine should be given 30 days prior to breeding. This type comes in combination with Lepto and other vaccines and is easier to administer, but it must be used according to directions if it is to be effective.

Bulls infected with vibrio have been cleared by use of two doses (of 5 ml) of the oil base vaccine, 30 days apart. All bulls should be vaccinated and given an annual booster in the fall. All cows in multiple owner herds and in herds adding used cows or bulls should be vaccinated. Lepto: May cause abortion and illness. It has not been commonly diagnosed in Utah in recent years, but is very difficult to diagnose. It is spread through urine and water contamination so is a potential threat to almost all cattle. It may also be carried by other species including rodents, dogs, swine and man.

Trichomoniasis: A common disease in Utah that causes early embryonic death. A vaccine is available with an efficacy of about 50%. It should be considered for use in infected herds which are mixed with other during the breeding season. Two doses are required initially. The second (and the annual booster) should be given 30 days prior to the beginning of breeding.

Scours

Rota and Corona Virus: Two viral agents that are common in Utah herds and contribute to scours. They usually produce only mild disease signs by themselves, but become more severe when combined with stress or other agents. A vaccine is available for problem herds. It requires two doses the first year and the last dose should be given at least three weeks prior to the start of calving. It may be used in combination with E. coli.

Coli (Coliform): A bacterial cause of scours that usually appears in calves under 5 days of age. A common contaminant in manure and may build up to epidemic levels. A vaccine requiring one or two initial doses is available for the cows prior to calving. A monoclonal antibody product is also available for use on calves at birth (by mouth) if a serious outbreak occurs in calves from dams that have not been vaccinated. It will provide some immediate, but short term protection.

Pinkeye

An eye infection due to a specific bacteria, that is commonly carried by many normal cattle. A herd outbreak is often precipitated by eye irritation (dust, sunlight, etc.). The infection is readily spread to other animals by face flies. Several vaccines are now available. Since the immunity they stimulate is not very long-lasting, these vaccines should be administered in the spring just prior to the fly season. This will provide the greatest protection during summer, the period of greatest exposure.

Pathogenic Bacteria

Bacteria that cause disease are called pathogenic bacteria. Bacteria can cause diseases in humans, in other animals, and also in plants. Some bacteria can only make one particular host ill; others cause trouble in a number of hosts, depending on the host specificity of the bacteria. The diseases caused by bacteria are almost as diverse as the bugs themselves and include food poisoning, tooth ache anthrax, even certain forms of cancer. It is impossible to sum up all bacterial diseases and it would be pretty boring. The Infectious Diseases fact sheets gives brief descriptions of diseases, including infectious diseases. Some diseases are named after the organisms that cause them, or is it the other way round?

If you want to have a look at pathogenic bacteria under the microscope:

- View here pathogenic bacteria under the microscope which also describes their properties, as part of a course on medical microbiology. Some of the terms used here are explained in our exhibit on pathogenicity.
- More links to microscopic pictures can be found in the exhibit on Images of bacteria.

Some pathogenic bacteria have received disproportionate attention in the press, e.g. the 'flesh-eating bacteria', which in real life are called Streptococci. Indeed they can cause spectacular, but fortunately uncommon symptoms. In the press, pathogenic bacteria are sometimes represented as (deadly) dangerous enemies that lurk in the dark, unseen, ready to attack you. Although that is exaggerated some bacteria can be life treatening, for example *Legionella pneumoniae*, the causative of Legionnaire's disease. These bacteria survive in moist places like air conditioners or hot-water pipes.

Though potentially life treatening, bacterial infections do not kill all their victims. Some bacteria kill a high percentage of people infected (they have a so-called a high mortality rate), but their relatively inefficient rate of spreading makes up for that. Other bacteria spread very easily, but they don't kill many of the people they infect. Imagine what would happen with a pathogen that spread very fast, killed all its victims; it would soon have none left to infect, and would die out together with the species on which it had been dependent. Bacterial pathogens don't eradicate their hosts completely. Although a popular theme for thrillers, this is a 'mission impossible' in real life.

When an infectious disease spreads around an area, and the cases of new infections reach a certain number, we call it an epidemic. Read about epidemics or visit the Epidemics Home Site. If, on the other hand, a certain disease is always present in low numbers of cases in a given area, that disease is said to be endemic in that area. Some epidemics become wide-spread and quickly reach distant parts of the world: in modern times people travel fast and frequent, and our bacteria travel with us. A classical example of such a pandemic (in this case caused by a virus) was a new type of influenza ("Spanish 'flu") that reached continent after continent early twentieth century, killing thousands of people on it's way. Although only a small proportion of the infected people died (the virus had a low mortality) so many people got infected that even the small proportion of deaths amounted to large numbers.

An epidemic or pandemic can only occur if the population is not immune to that disease. Read our special feature file on the history of infectious diseases about the times that pathogens could spread unlimited. Our exhibit on our immune system explains how immunity can prevent disease.

So why do epidemics occur? Either because they are caused by diseases that did not exist before, like AIDS, caused by the HIV virus, or because new variants of bacteria (or viruses) arrive in an area where they were not endemic before. This is why epidemics of the common 'flu' occur frequently: the virus causing influenza is able to change itself sufficiently to bypass our immunity built up from prior infections. Although not caused by bacteria, this site on influenza is very interesting if you want to understand epidemics of infectious diseases. Whenever a new virus type arises, there is the potential for a new epidemic. Fortunately, most of these new types are not as vicious as the Spanish 'flu. The experts are currently keeping an eye on bird flu, a strain of influenza that has not (yet?) learned to jump from person-to-person. If that would happen, a new pandemic could be the result.

An example of a bacterial disease that caused successive epidemics, and even pandemics, in recent times is *Vibrio cholerae*, the cause of cholera. Epidemiology is the study to establish the cause of a disease.

- Read this classic of cholera in London in the last century: an epidemiological 'whodunit' with John Snow as the chief inspector.

- Another classic epidemic in history was small pox raging through Europe in the 14th Century. Read our special feature file on the Black Death.

Bacteria have invented many different strategies to make us ill. These strategies, called bacterial pathogenicity, are the subject of an important division of medical microbiology. Understanding how certain bacteria make us ill can result in better treatment, vaccination, or prevention of that infectious disease. In another exhibit some of the common mechanisms of bacterial pathogenicity are explained. In order to keep this information balanced, now that you know what pathogenic bacteria are, why not also check out how commensal bacteria are good for you. You take healthy animals and often very quickly after you vaccinate, you can see simple things like itching of the skin or excessive licking of the paws, sometimes even with no eruptions. We see a lot of epilepsy, often after a rabies vaccination. Or dogs or cats can become aggressive for several days. Frequently, you'll see urinary tract infections in cats, often within three months after their [annual] vaccination. If you step back, open your mind and heart, you'll start to see patterns of illness post-vaccination."

Bloat and Torsion

"Bloat" or torsion of the stomach is sudden and often fatal. It can occur to any healthy large breed dog. Bloat is a condition where the stomach organ has twisted, cutting off vital functioning. It only happens in big dogs. The disease of bloat and torsion manifests itself under stressful conditions: vaccine, drug, anesthesia reactions and commercial kibble or canned food.

My German Shepheard dog, Kuuma, gets hit by this "bloat", or stomach spams once a month or so. It usually hits him soon after he eats kibbles (never when he eats only raw food - I feed him rawfood and kibbles because 100% raw gives him diarrheat) . Occasionally after he eats, he wakes up extremely agitated and restless, and tries to nibble on just about anything. It is obvious that he's in great pain. One thing that helps him, is to let him eat plenty of grass. He'll be grazing for 20 min or longer non-stop. If no grass is available, I let him eat wheatgrass which I grow in trays by the windowsill (I drink wheatgrass juice everyday). I have step by step instructions how to grow wheatgrass in apartments or homes. I believe that Kuuma would actually die if no grass was available for him to eat.

"Tragic middle-of-the-night trip to the emergency clinic, stomach the size of a basketball, turned upside-down. All they found in his stomach was kibble. I had suspected for a long time that something was wrong with his digestion. His stomach was always so noisy, he was always burping and farting. And the diarrhea! He was unable to digest and absorb commercial food. The kibble connection is a strong factor in bloat cases. He is now on a completely raw, whole food diet (BARF for Bones And Raw Foods). I've done a great deal of investigating, and have found out that it is VERY uncommon for dogs on the raw diets to bloat.

As far as I can tell, the best prevention for bloat is a raw whole food diet, done properly, of course. There are countless other benefits of the raw diet as well. There are many problems with the cooked diets that most people feed their dogs— the first being that the food is *cooked* and any enzymes have been killed, along with much nutritional value. Then there's the whole issue of very suspicious ingredients in commercial foods, significant toxins, and the fact that it's all got a very high percentage of grain. And the fats, once they're heated, turn into harmful trans fatty acids."

Nutrition: Is it Factor in Bloat and Torsion?

"It has been my experience that the number of incidents of bloat/ torsion have dropped dramatically over the past few years probably due to better quality meat based foods and the incorporation of whole foods, probiotics and digestive enzymes into the diet. I base this comment on the fact that I have had very few calls regarding bloat and torsion in 4+ years. Before that, I would average 2-3 calls for assistance per week. It is because of this experience and my interest in the prevention of disease through quality nutrition that has made me consider taking a closer look at the effects diet can have on the cause and prevention of bloat and torsion."

Leaky Gut Syndrome and Toxic Gut Syndrome can be the silent killers behind the cause for Bloat/Torsion and the misery of allergies. In this article I would like to explore what happens when a system is overrun with toxic levels of fungus, also known as yeast and high levels of pathogenic (bad) bacteria. Candida Albicans is a Fungus/ Yeast and a common microorganism that lives in the gut. But when there is an "overgrowth" of this fungus/yeast in the gut, it is called a systemic yeast infection, and it affects the health and well being of the whole animal or human. When on antibiotics or stressed, the pH balance of the gut is out of balance, and beneficial bacteria in the gut may be destroyed, and this insidious fungus and/or other pathogenic bacteria can take over and this overgrowth is very detrimental to our health and well being.

Sissy McGill knew many dog owners who had experienced the bloat problem in their animals. Sissy became interested in pet nutrition in 1974 after three of her Great Danes died of "bloat," a canine digestive problem. She learned that "bloat" was a common cause of death for dogs in the USA, but that the German vocabulary did not even assign a word for "bloat." Additionally, Tufts University research at the time revealed that "only in the USA do dogs die of bloat." It also suspected that the reason could be the corn, wheat, and soy in their diet. [Ed. Note – Interesting, since even people can get bloat from corn, wheat, and soy.] Europeans feed their dogs a natural type of food that doesn't contain the animal fat and soybean products.

In 1975, Sissy introduced the first all-natural dog food in the USA, containing no salt, animal fat, sugar-beet pulp, fillers, by-products, artificial flavours, colours, preservatives, corn, soy, or wheat – the last three being the top allergens in dogs. Learn how the Food and Drug Administration (FDA) relentlessly harassed her for selling animal products made from all natural ingredients. She ended up in jail. * Naturally relieve unpleasant symptoms of flatulence and gas in pets:

*   Reduce bloating, abdominal cramps and colic
*   Maintain digestive health and help with the symptoms of digestive disorders, including diarrhea and constipation.

Veterinary Medicine

Several diet-related factors were associated with a higher incidence of bloat. These include feeding only dry food, or feeding a single large daily meal. Dogs fed dry foods containing fat among the first four ingredients had a 170 percent higher risk for developing bloat. Dogs fed dry foods containing citric acid and were moistened prior to feeding had a 320 percent higher risk for developing bloat. Conversely, feeding a dry food containing a rendered meat-and-bone meal decreased risk by 53 percent in comparison with the overall risk for the dogs in the study. Mixing table food or canned food into dry food also decreased the risk of bloat.

During the past 30 years there has been a 1,500 percent increase in the incidence of bloat, and this has coincided with the increased feeding of dry dog foods. There is a much lower incidence of bloat in susceptible breeds in Australia and New Zealand. Feeding practices in these countries have been found to be less dependent on dry foods.

Dr. T.J. Dunn D.V.M. "There is ample proof that today's pet dogs and cats do not thrive on cheap, packaged, corn-based pet foods. Dogs and cats are primarily meat eaters; to fill them up with grain-based processed dry foods that barely meet minimum daily nutrient requirements has proven to be a mistake."

This parasite is a source of great anxiety among dog caretakers. Thanks in large part to the scare tactics of many veterinarians in promoting preventive drugs, many people believe that contracting heartworms is the equivalent of a death sentence for their dogs. This is not true.

I practiced for seven years in the Santa Cruz, California area, and treated many dogs with heartworms. The only dogs that developed symptoms of heart failure were those that were being vaccinated yearly, eating commercial dog food, and getting suppressive drug treatment for other symptoms, such as skin problems. My treatment, at that time, consisted of switching to a natural (that is, homemade) diet, stopping drug treatment whenever possible, and eliminating any chemical exposure, such as flea and tick poisons. I would usually prescribe hawthorn tincture as well. None of these dogs ever developed any symptoms of heart failure. (danger of: vaccines, commercial petfood, and antibiotics)

I concluded from this that it was not the heartworms that caused disease, but the other factors that damaged the dogs' health to the point that they could no longer compensate for an otherwise tolerable parasite load. It is not really that different from the common intestinal roundworms, in that most dogs do not show any symptoms. Only a dog whose health is compromised is unable to tolerate a few worms.

Furthermore, a truly healthy dog would not be susceptible to either type of worm in the first place.

It seems to me that the real problem is that allopathic attitudes have instilled in many of us a fear of disease, fear of pathogens and parasites, fear of rabies, as if these are evil and malicious entities just waiting to lay waste to a naive and unprotected public. Disease is not caused by viruses or by bacteria or by heartworm-bearing mosquitoes. Disease comes from within, and one aspect of disease can be the susceptibility to various pathogens. So the best thing to do is to address those susceptibilities on the deepest possible level, so that the pathogens will no longer be a threat. Most importantly, don't buy into the fear.

That having been said, there are practical considerations of risk versus benefit in considering heartworm prevention. The risk of a dog contracting heartworms is directly related to geographic location. In heavily infested areas the risk is higher, and the prospect of using a preventive drug more justifiable. Whatever you choose to do, a yearly blood test for heartworm microfilaria is important.

There are basically three choices with regard to heartworm prevention: drugs, nosodes, or nothing. There are currently a variety of heartworm preventive drugs, most of which are given monthly. I don't like any of them due to their toxicity, the frequency of side effects, and their tendency to antidote homeopathic remedies. Incidentally, the once-a-month preventives should be given only every 6 weeks.

The next option is the heartworm nosode. It has the advantage of at least not being a toxic drug. It has been in use it for over 10 years now, and I am reasonably confident that it is effective. It is certainly very safe. The biggest problem with the nosode is integrating it with homeopathic treatment. But at least it's less of a problem than with the drugs.

The last option, and in my opinion the best, is to do nothing. That is to say, do nothing to specifically prevent heartworm, but rather to minimise the chances of infestation by helping your dog to be healthier, and thereby less susceptible. This means avoiding those things that are detrimental to health, feeding a high quality homemade diet, regular exercise, a healthy emotional environment, and, most of all, constitutional homeopathic treatment. Of course, this will not guarantee that your dog will not get heartworms, but, under these conditions, even the worst-case scenario isn't so terrible. If your dog were to get heartworms, s/he shouldn't develop any symptoms as a result. For what it's worth, I never gave my dog any type of heartworm preventive, even when we lived in the Santa Cruz area where heartworms were very prevalent. I tested him yearly, and he never had a problem.

Dogs love Dr. Miller's Detox Tea too! Dogs enjoy drinking Dr. Miller's Detox Tea because it helps improve their digestion, thus eliminate bad breath and body odors. The tea also helps flush toxins and assists in cleansing waste and compacted fecal matter from the colon learn more.

An animal with a healthy immune system will be less likely to become infected with dog worms, including heartworm. Mosquitoes are less likely to bite healthy dogs. In addition, the healthy animals own defence system is able to kill off the larvae of any heartworm that may enter the bloodstream, thus preventing them from reaching maturity and causing harm. Factors that will weaken your dog's immune system include frequent vaccination, commercial pet foods, incorrect diet, stress and even conventional heartworm and other synthetic medication.

Fish Oil Helps Dogs with Lymphoma Live Longer

A diet supplemented with fish oil and the amino acid arginine appears to increase survival time in dogs with lymphoma, a cancer that affects white blood cells. Dogs with this kind of cancer, similar to non-Hodgkin's lymphoma in humans, are easily treated, but as with humans, their cancer tends to return.

Half of the dogs received a special chow with the two supplements in it, and the other half ate chow with soybean oil added. The two chows were identical in nutritional value, and formulated to be equally tasty to the dogs. All the dogs were being treated with the anti-cancer drug doxorubicin every three weeks, and were living at home with their owners.

Previous research has shown that some polyunsaturated fatty acids, like those found in fish oil, may help prevent the growth and spread of cancer tumours, and may help prevent cachexia — the devastating weight loss and muscle wasting seen in some cancer patients despite adequate nutrition. Likewise, arginine supplements have been reported to improve immune responses, and might help the body fight cancer.

The dogs were fed one of the chows twice a day during and after their cancer treatment. The researchers report that compared to the control dogs, those who ate the supplemented chow showed higher blood levels of two fatty acids called C20:5 and C22:6 that seem particularly effective in fighting cancer. Dogs with more of these fatty acids in their blood also tended to have more normal levels of lactic acid, which tends to accumulate in the blood when metabolism is disrupted in cancer patients.

The dogs with higher levels of these two fatty acids survived longer than those with lower levels, and had longer remissions, periods of time before their disease came back.

Did you know that the root cause of serious chronic diseases such as heart disease, Alzheimer's disease, cancer, arthritis, and asthma has been identified as chronic inflammation? Although numerous studies have confirmed these findings, few physcians are aware of or consider the fact that the battle against inflammation is at the forefront of the fight for health and well-being of the global population. Authors Joseph Maroon and Jeffrey Bost have set out to reverse that trend with "Fish Oil: The Natural Anti-Inflammatory." For years dog health supplies have included toxic materials to artificially maintain dog health as a temporary measure. The time has come to change to a more natural approach toward dog health. Natural remedies have been shown to achieve more immediate, more complete and longer lasting health, vitality, quality and longevity of dogs lives.

Hypertrophic Osteodystrophy (HOD)

Hypertrophic osteodystrophy causes lameness and extreme pain in young growing dogs, usually of a large breed. Great danes, German shepherds, dobermans, retrievers and weimaraners are examples of breeds that may be affected by this condition. It appears to occur in weimaraners as a vaccine reaction and this may also affect mastiffs and great Danes. In this case, it usually occurs a few days after vaccination and may appear to be worse than the "average" case on radiographs.

HOD usually shows up as an acute lameness, often seeming to affect all four legs simultaneously. Affected dogs may stand in a "hunched up" stance or refuse to stand up at all. They may have a fever but this is not consistently present. They usually have painful swellings around the lower joints on the legs. Some puppies will die from this disease, some suffer permanent disability but many recover later. The disease is so painful that many owners elect to euthanize the puppy rather than watch it suffer, despite the reasonably good chance for recovery, long term. Affected dogs may be so ill that they refuse to eat. If your dog has been on certain antibiotics 2-12 days before your puppy exhibited HOD like symptoms, then it is possible the dog is having an antibiotic reaction and not HOD.

Correctly prescribed homeopathic remedies can often undue the damage caused by vaccines Homeopathy is noted for its success to antidote or remove the toxic effects of vaccines and to re-establish balance in the organism and restore health. Certain homeopathic remedies can minimise vaccine damage. A professional homeopathic vet should be consulted for more information.

Causes, Predisposing Factors and Treatment

Dee Blanco, D.V.M - "You take healthy animals and often very quickly after you vaccinate, you can see simple things like itching of the skin or excessive licking of the paws, sometimes even with no eruptions. We see a lot of epilepsy/seizure, often after a rabies vaccination. Or dogs or cats can become aggressive for several days. Frequently, you'll see urinary tract infections in cats, often within three months after their annual vaccination. If you step back, open your mind and heart, you'll start to see patterns of illness post-vaccination." Health Hazard of Routine Vaccination: placing our animals at risk

Some dogs are sensitive to chemicals and if you feed and water them from a plastic bowl, they ingest some of the chemicals and it can help induce the seizures. There has been reports of a reduction of seizures when the immune system was modulated and the inflammation reduced with Transfer Factor.

Magnesium Deficiency and Your Animal's Health

Holistic veterinarian Roger DeHaan, DVM states that some forms of epilepsy respond to supplementation of vitamin B6, magnesium, and manganese. Learn more about magnesium deficiency in people and animals

William Pollak D.V.M. - "The most common direct cause of seizures seen in clinical practice in our pets is parasitic infection combined with nutritional deficiencies based on 100% commercial pet food feeding." Animal Epilepsy/Seizure - Causes, Predisposing Factors and Treatment.

"Feeding a natural raw food diet is vital to not only maintaining the health of your pet, but also keeping ideal immune function alive and well. Many times after eliminating seizures through improving the diet, seizures return after commercial pet food is re-instituted. "

"Today's modern approach to dealing with these problems is the administration of more chemicals, injectable or otherwise and even greater processed "prescription" diets. Seizures are masked by giving chemicals that profoundly dull the CNS, slowing it down and confusing it so as to reduce the likelihood of another seizure. These chemicals oftentimes do not work and further confuse the biological system as already described earlier. The underlying imbalance is not directly addressed. Deranged metabolic disorders due to chemical shortages or imbalances are superficially addressed by further limitations in the diet; i.e.even more severely processed foods."

Here is another network that provides additional information on canine epilepsy and other diseases that cause seizures in dogs including canine hypothyroidism. Their canine epilepsy section provides information about canine epilepsy, what happens when your dog has a seizure, possible causes of seizures by age, what tests are used to diagnose canine epilepsy, and information from our Guardian Angels on what they would do differently "if they knew then what they know now." Under medications you will find information a number of medications that are used to control seizures in dogs. Those medications include the more commonly used Phenobarbital and Potassium Bromide as well as newer drugs such as Gabapentin and Felbamate. The section on thyroid contains several articles on canine hypothyroidism and the connection between low thyroid and seizures.

Fulvic Acid Nature's Poison Detoxifier

Fulvic acid acts as an important protective agent. An important aspect of humic substances is related to their sorptive interaction with environmental chemicals, either before or after they reach concentrations, toxic to living organisms. 33 The toxic herbicide know as Paraquat is rapidly detoxified by humic substances (fulvic acid). 34 Fulvic acids have a special function with respect to the demise of organic compounds applied to soil as pesticides. As the most powerful, natural electrolyte known, fulvic acid restores electrical balance to damaged cells, neutralises toxins and can eliminate food poisoning within minutes. When it encounters free radicals with unpaired positive or negative electrons, it supplies an equal and opposite charge to neutralise the free radical. Fulvic acid acts as a refiner and transporter of organic materials and cell nutrients. According to A. Szalay, fulvic acid has the ability to dramatically detoxify herbicides, pesticides, and other poisons that it interacts with – this includes many radioactive elements. This detoxification process may extend to animals and humans, since we are the end-users of these plants.

"Over the years, I began to pull this herb and that herb out of the book, such as the wonderful use of RAW CUCUMBER JUICE topically for CONJUNCTIVITIS, the use of GARLIC internally and externally for ALL TYPES OF PARASITES. I began to use herbal immune tonics, heart tonics, liver cleansers and arthritis herbs. Each year I picked herbs like fruit from a great bearing fruit tree. Whatever I wanted the tree seemed to have for me. All my instincts told me I had stumbled upon the Great Cornucopia of Cure."

The Pet Parasite Cleanse

Pets have many of the same parasites that we get, including Ascaris (common roundworm), hookworm, Trichinella, Strongyloides, heartworm and a variety of tapeworms. Every pet living in your home should be deparasitized (cleared of parasites) and maintained on a parasite program. Monthly trips to your vet are not sufficient. You may not need to get rid of your pet to keep yourself free of parasites. But if you are ill it is best to board it with a friend until you are better. Your pet is part of your family and should be kept as sweet and clean and healthy as yourself This is not difficult to achieve.

Glyconutrients/Saccharides in Veterinary Medicine

Arthur Young DVM, a Certified Homeopathic Veterinarian, uses glyconutrients in his practice on all animals from birds to horses. He always advises his clients to add glyconutrients to their pets diet. Decades of consuming nutritionally questionable commercial pet food products, the proven harmful effects of over vaccination, combined with the unfortunate dependency on steroids and antibiotics have, according to many reliable sources greatly contributed to a national decline in animal health.

The innate ability of the body to heal itself has been seriously compromised in many animals, particularly dogs, cats, and horses. Glyconutrients are compatible with any type of treatment prescribed by both conventional and alternative practitioners. These essential carbohydrates strengthen the body's inner environment which, in turn, enhances the energy that stimulates the immune system, as well as a process called "cell communication". This communication network results in all of the organs working with one another in an orderly sequence of body reactions. Without these activities, good health is impossible to attain. Although the formulation is produced for human consumption, holistic veterinarians have also recognised the importance of glyconutrients in supporting the handling of health challenges in animals. Credit goes to Günter Blobel, M.D., Ph.D. (Rockefeller

University), winner of the 1999 Nobel Prize for Medicine "for the discovery that (glyco) proteins have intrinsic signals that govern their transport and localisation in the cell."

Guinea Pigs, Hamsters, Rabbits Holistic Health and Nutrition

Many rabbit owners and lovers are not aware that natural care and holistic health treatments are available for their pet, and that it can be extremely effective in a variety of conditions. Rabbits have a rapid metabolism and respond well to treatment modalities such as acupuncture, homeopathy and flower remedies. The other benefit of using such therapies is that there are very few, if any side effects, unlike a lot of drugs such as antibiotics, which rabbits tend to be very sensitive to.

Ferrets Natural Health Care and Optimum Diet

To maintain optimum health, ferrets require a diet which most closely resembles that which they would get in the wild. They also require some sunlight. Ferrets are strict carnivores, meaning they are designed to eat whole prey items, which includes all parts of the killed animal.

Because of the short GI tract and the poor absorption of nutrients, ferrets require a diet that is highly concentrated with FAT as the main source of calories (energy) and highly digestible MEAT-BASED PROTEIN. The bottom line is that ferrets use fat for energy not carbohydrates and they need a highly digestible meat-based protein not vegetable protein. The most appropriate diet for a ferret would be whole prey foods such as rats, mice or chicks. The worst examples of processed diets are the ferret treat foods

Domesticated Animals (including ferrets and rodents) Suffer from Minerals and Vitamin Deficiency

Our soil, plants, and especially commercial foods are woefully deficient in key nutrients. Scientists theorise that mineral deficiency subjects us, and our animals, to more diseases, aging, sickness and destruction of our physical well-being than any other factor in personal health. Domesticated ferrets, like our domesticated dogs and cats, are prone to suffer from minerals and trace mineral deficiency which makes them prone to diseases. A good source of naturally occuring trace minerals and vitamins for ferrets and other pets are:

Marine Phytoplankton

Dr. Jerry Tennant, M.D. says that marine phytoplankton contains almost everything one needs to sustain life and to restore health by providing the raw materials to make new cells that function normally. Marine phytoplankton has been called "the most nutritionally dense foods on the planet". Containing a wide range of trace elements, amino acids, vitamins, minerals, chlorophyll, enzymes and cellular materials, marine phytoplankton promotes and maintains optimum health by boosting and supporting all systems within the body.

Seaweed (kelp). Sea Vegetables (Spirulina - Kelp - Chlorella) have been acknowledged as a detoxifyer, a balanced nourishment and a miraculous healing plant. Ocean / Sea algae are the richest natural source of minerals, trace minerals and rear earth elements.

Fulvic minerals consist of an immense arsenal and array of naturally occuring powerful phytochemicals, biochemicals, supercharged antioxidants, free-radical scavengers, super oxide dismutases, nutrients, enzymes, hormones, amino acids, antibiotics, antivirals, and antifungals

Bee Pollen contains all the essential components of life. The percentage of rejuvenating elements in bee pollen remarkably exceeds those present in brewer's yeast and wheat germ. Bee pollen corrects the deficient or unbalanced nutrition, common in the customs of our present-day civilization of consuming incomplete foods.

Flaxoil: holistic veterinarians are beginning to recommend to their clients that they supplement their animals diet with a daily dose of flaxseed oil and other nutrients for optimum health and vitality. The vets are finding remarkable results in clearing up skin conditions, relieving arthritic and inflammatory pain, as well as improved over all pet health. (Suzie Zeeman gives flaxoil to her ferrets. She says that their fur looks shinny and thick, and feels soft and smooth since on flaxoil.)"

Bentonite and Pascalite clay: It has helped cows with scours and pneumonia. Veterinarians use it on dogs, cats, horses, etc... for various afflictions including injuries and infections. Pets are helped, too.

Transfer Factor Plus - Canine and Feline Formulas are advanced immune support supplements formulated or dogs and cats (also good for ferrets). According to veterinarians, the powerful and proprietary blend of ingredients work together to activate and enhance the immune system's ability to respond to the many pathogens may pets come into contact with.

Barley Dog is the original "green" supplement made from the juice of organic Barley grass with a hickory smoked flavor. It provides active enzymes, vitamins C and E, beta-carotene, amino acids, chlorophyll, proteins and essential trace minerals. Regular use can promote healthy skin and coat, reduce bad breath, improve digestion and restore energy levels.

Cindy Engles, Ph.D., documents that for millennia humans have observed animals in the wild eating plants and minerals and applying naturally occurring topical antitoxins from the same sources to combat infectious wounds, parasites and internal disorders. Herds of elephants risk injury and death in a perilous journey to hidden salt caves where they supplement their sodium deficient diet. Monkeys rub poisonous millipedes on their fur to repel biting, disease-carrying insects. Birds line their nests with parasite-resistant herbs. Engel details a world where nature is the pharmacy and every animal is its own practitioner.

On page 83 of Wild Health Cindy Engles, Ph.D. also explains why animals eat their own feces. "Eating feces (coprophagy) is one way animals such as gorillas, elephants, rabbits, and hares add to their supply of essential bacteria through adult life. It is therefore an important aspect of their health care. Overzealous rabbit owners could inadvertently cause disease in their pets by cleaning out the droppings too quickly. By reingesting their own soft pellets (and discarting the hard, dry ones), rabbits extract further nutrients from their food and obtain essential vitamins made in the gut by microorganism."

A chimp with a stomach ache may seek out a broad-spectrum antidote like the bitter-leaf. Or it may swallow whole leaves from several different kinds of hairy plants: leaves with 'Velcro' hooks help clear out intestinal worms. Bears before hibernation and snow geese before migration also turn to Velcro plants. Domestic dogs and cats chew grass, which has the same scouring effect. Many wild animals, and some people, develop 'pica' when ill, a craving to eat earth - particularly clay, which assuages diarrhoea and binds to many plant poisons. Among the most famous clay-eaters are the parrots of the Amazon.

Scarlet macaws, blue and gold macaws, and hosts of smaller birds perch together in their hundreds to excavate the best clay layer along a riverbank. Parrots' regular diet is tree seeds, which the trees defend with toxic chemicals, Canine autoimmune haemolytic anaemia is an autoimmune disease in dogs where the red blood cells are damaged or destroyed by the animal's own antibodies, resulting in anaemia. Haemolysis may take place within the blood vessels or in the spleen. In addition to haemolysis, permanent or intermittent inactivity of the bone marrow is common. According to information contained on the leaflet accompanying the Rabdomun rabies vaccine, extraneous proteins found in some vaccines can cause autoimmune disease.

Aromatherapy

Aromatherapy is the art and science of using from plant sources for health and wellbeing. Essential oils have a potentially powerful healing capacity. The early civilizations — Egyptian, Greek, Roman, Chinese, Egyptian, — made use of aromatic plant materials in religious ritual and to promote physical and mental wellness.

Hilary Jupp, a former breeder of Wolfhounds, is now a judge for the breed at championship show level. Her main interests (besides Irish wolfhounds!) are in the field of nutrition and holistic therapies for animals. She is a bio-energy therapist, a Reiki Master, has a Doctorate in Radionic Medicine, and is especially interested in channelling, animal communication, flower essences, and homoeopathy. She has written the Breed notes for the British weekly paper *"Dog World"* since 1986, has written for it on natural therapies, and for several years wrote for Hoflin Publishing's *"Irish Wolfhound Quarterly"* and *"Windhound"*. In her wonderful web site you will find of information about alternative therapies for animals such as:

Acupressure, Bio Energy Therapy, Bowen Technique, Chiropractic, Massage, Osteopathy, Tellington Ttouch, and Animal Links. Hilary also list various natural treatments for various conditions

Acupuncture was first used to treat animals over 3000 years ago in Asia. An elephant had a stomach disorder similar to bloating. The healer used slender needles placed in specific positions on the skin to relieve the pain and to help the elephant. Since that time acupuncture has been used all over the world to alleviate many kinds of health problems for many species of animals.

Temperament and Behavioural Problems, Cancer, Epileptiform fits, Heart disease, Digestive disorders, Skin disorders, Bone and joint disorders and more.

- Preventing and Healing Animal Cancer, arthritis, and other disease with flaxoil
- Amazing Healing Clay: a wonderful nutritional supplement for animals
- Orthomolecular/Nutritional Medicine for Animals
- For Cats and Dogs' Optimum Health: Sprouting and Grasses
- Adding Kelp meal to your pet's diet to promote optimum health

- Ready to Eat Health-Food For Your Pet: commercial prepared, ready-to-eat frozen or freeze dried RAW meals for dogs, cats and ferrets. (if homemade food is not feasable).

"For a return to health, pets require a diet which strengthens the immune system and most closely resembles that which they would get in the wild".

Frustrated with the Failures of Conventional Veterinary Medicine: "After 10 years of traditional veterinary practice I became tired of having no treatment for chronic disease, incurable conditions, and a plethora of allergic maladies which seem to plague all veterinary practices. I was frustrated with giving animals cortisone because I had no other solutions, or using antibiotics for infections which I knew were of viral origin.

Amazing animal health improvements and cures of cancer and other chronic disease with natural, alternative health care and optimum nutrition.

This is a list of professional holistic veterinarians and animal consultants who are willing to offer phone consultations. (If there are no holistic veterinarians in your hometown, phone consultations for homeopathic treatment can be just as effective as an office consultation, especially if you already have a diagnosis of your animal's condition.)

This is a group where sharing of information on the application of homeopathy (for people and animals) is given in a practical, usable format.

Dedicated to the herbal, natural, alternative, and holistic care and keeping of livestock, animals and pets. Dedicated to the herbal, natural, alternative, and holistic care and keeping of livestock, animals and pets. Great for small farm owners and homesteaders. Although goats are my first love, we raise and chat about all sorts of animals from the farm.

This is a list whereby all who are interested in healing with herbs and natural methods can voice their opinions and share their views. The predominant theme is "Herbal Remedies" and "Natural Healing" for you goats. We welcome the discussion of other animals but the list is primarily directed at alternatives or supplementing for your caprine friends. This is for seeking other ways , i.e.. Alternatives and/ or supplementation to conventional medicine for those who would like to seek other methods of naturally raising their stock. It is not restricted to Classical Homeopathy, and may , to a degree, include adjuncts such as diet + nutrition, herbs, lifestyle etc., and health related topics such as vaccination etc.

This list will contain information pertaining to dog health (both in pure breeds and mixed breeds of all ages), primarily with regards to drugs that can or have caused illness and/or death in dogs. The focus is presently on the drug Rimadyl (carprofen). However, all issues regarding dogs' health can be addressed at this site. Only those genuinely concerned and seriously committed to the welfare of dogs are encouraged to join the list.

For Veterinarians and for those with care of pets and animals. For pet owners: Introduction to Veterinary Homeopathy. The Elizabethan collar is a type of plastic collar that is effective in preventing pets from licking or biting themselves. The only time I will use such collar is to prevent my animal from tearing up surgical sutures, until healing is complete. I will never use such collar to prevent my dog or cat from licking skin eruptions, hot spots, or inflammed and infected area on their bodies. The built in germicide found in the saliva of a dog or a cat amazingly heals wounds in record time. Any injuries are carefully licked and coated with antiseptic saliva from the tongue. This aids in preventing infection entering into a wound.

Natural Herbal Digestive Aids for Dogs and Cats

"Most of what I've learned about the holistic care and treatment of my dog I've learned from Shirley's Wellness Cafe. This vast and detailed resource is the result of a journey of natural healing that webmaster Shirley used on herself and her family to completely turn their lives around. Those lessons are applied here with full force for the benefit of our canine companions. Raw food diets, detailed feature articles on a wide variety of wellness topics, health reports, and studies are all represented here in a slightly cluttered, yet home-style approach that blends a first-person knowledge and passion for the subject with a caring and nurturing writing style. Thank you, Shirley. The 'net's a better place because of sites like yours

Animal Husbandry and Cattle Management in *Arthasastra*

Humans had to interact closely with nature for their basic needs since prehistoric times; their daily life was totally dependent on plants and animals. Thus the relationship between humans and animal is very ancient. *Atharvaveda* has several references to dairy farming, cattle health care etc. Asoka, the Buddhist emperor (300BC), established a network of veterinary hospitals throughout India.

Kautilyayys *Arthasastra* (321-296 BC) describes a well-managed animal husbandry and cattle management system. In this article I have dealt with ancient animal husbandry from the *Arthasastrayy*s point of view.

We are amazed at the detailed and scientific regulations for seemingly such a minor activity 2300 years back. It also shows the concern of the state not only to exploit the animals but also to live with them symbiotically. Large cattle-sheds were well regulated, and so were the wild game sanctuaries where animals were safe from poaching. Even for animals, a medical ethics was enforced by *Arthasastra*.

Let us first introduce Kautilya and his *Arthasastra*. All sources of Indian traditions -Brahmanical, Buddhist and Jain - agree that Kautilya destroyed the Nanda dynasty and installed Chandragupta Maurya on the throne of Magadha. The name Kautilya denotes that he was of the Kutila gotra. The name yyChanakyayy means that he was the son of Chanaka, though yyVishnuguptayy was his personal name. *Arthasastra* was composed by Kautilya in probably between 321-296 BC, though there are doubts about the date of the composition of *Arthasastra*. A workshop held by the Indian Council for Historical Research, Delhi, concluded that the *Arthasastra* in its present form was a compilation made by a scholar, Kautilya, in 150 AD.

But there is no doubt that Chandragupta Maurya ascended the throne around 321 BC. *Arthasastra* had never been forgotten in India, but the text itself was not available until, dramatically, a full text on palm leaf in the *grantha* script, along with a fragment of an old commentary by Bhattasvamin, came into the hands of Dr. R. Shamasastry of Mysore in 1904. And finally he published the text not only in Hindi but also in English in 1909. *Arthasastra* is a valuable document, which throws light on the state and society of India at c. 300 BC. Here we can say that Kautilyayys *Arthasastra* is totally an administrative text of ancient India, especially of the Mauryan times. Animal husbandry or cattle management was one of the main administrative jobs of the state. Kautilyayys *Arthasastra* also throws light on ancient cattle management practices of the country.

Animal Husbandry

Arthasastra contains an elaborate analysis regarding various aspects of livestock with prescriptions for their better management. Kautilya was also highly conscious about the benefits man gets from different species of animals. Both domestic and wild animals were well protected by all means in Kautilyayys time. Kautilya mentioned a variety of animals such as deer, bison, birds, fish, cattle, elephants, horses, asses, pigs, camels, sheep, goat, etc. According to *Arthasastra,* cattle rearing was the second most important economic activity. Cow and she-buffaloes were reared for milk and the bulls and he-buffaloes were used as drought animals. Ghee, which had the advantage of being easily stored and transported, was the main end product. Cheese was supplied to the army, buttermilk was fed to dogs and pigs and whey mixed with oilcake was used as animal feed. Wool was obtained from sheep and goats.

Cattle Superintendent and Cowherds

Crown herds were the responsibility of the chief superintendent who either employed cowherds, milkers, etc. on wages or gave some herds to a contractor. Chief superintendent was responsible for cattle (cows, bulls and buffaloes), goats, sheep, horses, donkeys, camels and pigs. He had to keep a record of every animal in the different types of herds, of the total of all such animals, of the number that die or are lost, the total collection of milk and ghee and other products. Private herds could also be entrusted to the state for protection on payment. Private owners of animals paid a sales tax of a quarter *pana* for every animal sold. The superintendent of cows had to supervise the maintenance of cows as well as bull, oxen, buffaloes, and their young calves.

The duties of a superintendent were: supervise herds and obtain exact information about abandoned and useless herds; maintain class of herds by registering each animalyys natural and branded marks, colour, and distance from one horn to another; update the number of stray cattle and register total number of cattle lost permanently; collection of information about total production of milk and ghee or clarified butter, etc.

The duties of cowherds were: graze their herds in forest grounds under suitable guards and in groups of ten according to their types; treat the animals during the period of their illness; take care of animals when animals went to river or lakes to drink water; to ensure that the watering place is safe and free of crocodiles and not muddy; to milk timely; inform the owners about the loss of cattle and cause of loss; to hang bells around the necks of timid animals in order to frighten snakes and to locate them easily when grazing; in rainy season, autumn and early winter, cows and she-buffaloes were to be milked twice a day and in late winter, spring and summer only once a day.

Generally four types of herd were recognised in the *Arthasastra*. Those:

- *Looked after by attendants:* - the chief superintendent employed, for each herd of 100 animals, one cowherd or buffalo herdsman, a milker, a churner and a hunter guard who would protect the herds from wild animals.

- *Looked after under contract:* - a balanced herd of 100 animals could be given to some one on contract.

- *Unproductive animals:* - a balanced herd of 100 animals may be given to someone for an annual payment, related to what the herd can produce.

- *Private cattle looked after for a share:* - private cattle owners could place their animals under the protection of the King on payment of a protection share.

Basically cowherds played an important role in the maintenance of livestock. On the other hand, the herdsmen had to pay one-tenth of dairy produce to the superintendent of cows. Therefore, such supervision was a source of royal income.

Official Breeder

Animal breeding was given special attention in Kautilyayys *Arthasastra*. The King appointed an official breeder for improving the breed of animals. According to *Arthasastra*, for breeding purpose, the following proportion of male animals should be kept for every herd of 100 animals:

Accounting of Animals

According to Kautilya, the Chief Superintendent should keep an account of the animals as follows:

- All calves should be identified (by branding or by nicking the ear) within a month or two of birth; all stray cattle be marked if they remain unclaimed for more than two mounts.

- Every animal should be identified in the records with the details of the branding mark, any natural identification marks, the colour, and peculiarity of horns.

- An account should be maintained of cattle lost.

Animal Welfare

There is extensive evidence in the *Arthasastra* about Kautilyayys concern for the welfare of animals. Regulations for the protection of wild life, a long list of punishment for cruelty to animals, rations for animals, rules for grazing and the responsibility of veterinary doctors are some of the major topics.

- Animal sanctuary was the remarkable feature of *Arthasastra*. As part of creation of the infrastructure of a settled and prosperous kingdom, an animal sanctuary, where all animals were welcomed as guests was established.

- Killing or injuring protected species and animals in reserved parks and sanctuaries was prohibited. Even animals, which had turned dangerous, were not to be killed within the sanctuary but had to be caught, taken outside and then killed.

- Sea fish which had strange or unusual characteristics, fresh water fish from lakes, rivers, tanks or canals; game birds or birds for pleasure such as curlew, osprey, swan, pheasant, partridge, parrot and mynah; and all auspicious birds and animals were declared as protected species.

- The chief protector did not allow the catching of fish, or the trapping, hurting or killing of animals whose slaughter was not customary.

- Live birds and deer received as tax were let loose in the sanctuaries.

- If protected animals or those from reserved forests strayed and were found grazing where they should not, they were to be driven away without hurting them. Stray cattle were to be driven off with rope or a whip without harming them.

- Butchers paid tax for sold meat at the rates given below:

Kautilya ordains that Butchers should follow some rules and regulations, like: should sell only freshly killed animals. The sale of swollen meat, rotten meat and meat from naturally dead animals was prohibited. Fish without head or bones should not be sold. Meat may be sold with or without bones. If sold with bones, equivalent compensation (for the weight of the bone) was to be given.

Grazing Places or Pastures

Pastures were basically required for grazing domestic cattle during ancient India when stall-feeding was rarely adopted. Pastures located in the forest were relieved from danger of tigers, beasts, and thieves. A separate clause was prescribed by Kautilya to protect livestock in pastures and defined the penalties for promoting imprudent grazing of pastures. Pasture lands within the village boundary were the responsibility of the village headman. He collected the charge for grazing on common land and ensured that cattle do not graze or stray into cultivated private fields or gardens or eat the grains in stored sheds. Headman had the responsibility for collecting the revenue for the village from the charges levied on grazing in common land, from the prescribed fines and the fines levied by the state.

According to *Arthasastra*, bulls belonging to village temples, stud bulls and cows up to ten days after calving were exempt from payments from the following grazing charges:

Healthcare of Animals

Kautilya set forth guidelines for providing medicine to livestock. Various mixtures were prescribed to cure different diseases. He maintained that cowherds shall apply remedies to calves or aged cows or cows suffering from diseases. Regarding the dosage he mentioned that proportion of a dose is as much as an *aksha* (quantity) to men; twice as much to cows and horses and four times as much to elephants and camels.

Kautilya had provided the facility of veterinary doctors, who were to cure the ill animals. But Kautilya fined the veterinary doctors when the condition of sick animals became worse. If the animal died they had to repay the cost of animal. We thus see that the medical ethics was already enforced by the state in ancient India.

Nutrition Management of Cattle

Kautilya had analysed many cattle problems and set the guidelines:

- Drought oxen would be provided with subsistence in proportion to the duration of service rendered.
- Milch cows would be provided with subsistence in proportion to the milk obtained from them.
- All cattle would be provided fodder and water abundantly.

Animal Products

Kautilya even standardised the purity of the animal products:

Ghee: Normal yield of ghee from 1 drona of milk:

Kurchika- Cheese (to be supplied to the army)

Kilata- Whey (mixed with oil cake, used as animal feed)

Butter-removed buttermilk- Not for human consumption, to be fed to dogs and pigs.

Such as hair, skins, bladder, bile, tendons, teeth, hooves and horns were useful products of wild animals form the forest.

Importance of Elephants and Horses

In *Arthasastra*, elephants and horses played a major role in defence practices. According to *Arthasastra,* the best army had best horses and elephants, of good pedigree, strength, youthfulness, vitality, loftiness, speed, mettle, good training, stamina, a lofty mien, obedience, auspicious marks, and good conduct. Kautilya categorised several kinds of elephants and their physical characteristics: war elephants, riding elephants, and untrainable elephants. The state took into account the physical characteristics of elephants with red patches, evenly fleshed, of even sides and rounded girth, with a curved backbone and well endowed with flesh. The following structure of army shows the importance of elephants and horses:

Small Animal Diseases

Louise Pasteur, a Frenchman who was neither a physician nor a veterinarian moved into the spotlight to help find a vaccine for Rabies. He began the study of Rabies when two rabid dogs were brought into his laboratory. One of the dogs suffered from the dumb form of the disease: his lower jaw hung down, he foamed at the mouth, and his eyes had a rather vacant look. The other dog was furious: he snapped, bit any object held out to him, and let out frightening howls (McCoy 65).

Through the studies already observed, rabies was transmitted through the bite of a rabid animal, and that the incubation period varied from a few days to several months. Beyond this, nothing definite was known.

Then M. Bouley, a professor of veterinary science, noted a germ or organism in the saliva of a rabid dog. Pasteur confirmed Bouley's findings by collecting some mucus from a child bitten by a rapid dog, and injecting it into rabbits.

The results of this experiment ended with all the rabbits dying within 36 hours. This experiment established two facts: an organism was present in the saliva of rabid animals, and it could be transmitted to another animal or a human being through a bite (McCoy 66).

Further research led Pasteur to the conclusion that the rabies organism was located in other parts of the infected animal's body besides its saliva. Experiments on the skulls of rabid dogs shoed that the brain contained the rabies virus. Pasture then cultured some viruses from several rabid dogs' brains. The virus was then injected into rabbits. In every case the rabies would appear within 14 days (McCoy 67).

After several experiments, Pasteur went on to perfect a rabies vaccine. He first demonstrated to physicians and veterinarians that the rabies could be cultured from the brains of living dogs.

Pasteur successfully proved that his antirabies vaccine could now be safely administered and animals could be vaccinated against the disease.

Chapter 6

Ethical Treatment of Animals

Ethical Treatment of Animals

The treatment of animals is all around us, we can watch television and we see it, it is in newspapers, on our computers as we browse, and we can even see bulletins as we walk down the street. Many different chains that are involved in animal cruelty are unknown to others, we can all start to wonder after some research has come before us to read. Then you can think about what you have bit into (literally) and swallowed.

"Fast food chains such as McDonald's, KFC, and Burger King are major players in the Production, marketing, and consumption of animal-derived food throughout the world".

In doing some research in August 22 ,2006 in the city of Chicago being the first to ban restaurants to sell foie gras, a delicacy prepared from goose liver. The gourmet delicacy is prepared by force-feeding ducks and geese to fatten their livers-often to the point of bursting. Force feeding fowl through a funnel inserted in their throats is a blatant example of animal cruelty(302 Business and Society Review).

According to the Business and Society Review little protection is afforded to animals raised for human consumption; they are subject to abuse throughout the process of production, transportation, and slaughter. Some of the worst examples of abuse are found in factory farms where animals may literally never see the light of day or be afforded enough space to even turn around.

A few specific examples that are noteworthy, critics of intensive animal farming contend:

Animals are often genetically altered to increase size and/or shorten growing times. In doing this workers make animals fat fast and give the hormones that make them grow bigger than normal size. Animals potentially have deformities and even death from this process.

Bovine Spongiform Encephalopathy

Bovine spongiform encephalopathy (BSE) is a relatively new disease found primarily in cattle. This disease of the bovine breed was first seen in the United Kingdom in November 1986 by histopathological examination of affected brains (Kimberlin, 1993). From the first discovery in 1986 to 1990 this disease developed into a large-scale epidemic in most of the United Kingdom, with very serious economic consequences (Moore, 1996).

BSE primarily occurs in adult cattle of both male and female genders. The most common age at which cows may be affected is between the ages of four and five (Blowey, 1991). Due to the fact that BSE is a neurological disease, it is characterised by many distinct symptoms: changes in mental state 'mad-cow', abnormalities of posture, movement, and sensation (Hunter, 1993). The duration of the clinical disease varies with each case, but most commonly lasts for several weeks. BSE continues to progress and is usually considered fatal (Blowey, 1991).

After extensive research, the pathology of BSE was finally determined. Microscopic lesions in the central nervous system that consist of a bilaterally symmetrical, non-inflammatory vacuolation of neuronal perikarya and grey-matter neuropil was the scientists' overall conclusion (Stadthalle, 1993). These lesions are consistent with the diseases of the more common scrapie family. Without further investigation, the conclusion was made that BSE was a new member of the scrapie family (Westgarth, 1994). Transmission of BSE is rather common throughout the cattle industry. After the incubation period of one to two years, experimental transmission was found possible by the injection of brain homogenates from clinical cases (Swanson, 1990). This only confirmed that BSE is caused by a scrapie-like infectious agent.

Seventy-percent of antibiotics used in the United States are fed to cattle, pigs, and chickens that have not shown disease symptoms, but rather receive the drugs prophylactically. This practice, known as nontherapeutic use (in contrast to therapeutic use of antibiotics for treating sick animals on an individual basis), has contributed significantly to the development of new strains of antibiotic resistant bacteria.

The diminished efficacy of these antibiotics poses an urgent public health concern for animals, humans, and for children in particular, who are especially susceptible to antibiotic resistant infections. New infections are constantly being linked to industrial farming, including Methicillin-resistant Staphylococcus aureus (MRSA), a disease causing 18,000 deaths each year in the U.S.

Representative Louise Slaughter (D-NY) and 46 House cosponsors and the late Senator Edward Kennedy (D-MA) and Senator Olympia Snowe (R-ME) and 3 Senate cosponsors moved to address this health threat through the Preservation of Antibiotics for Medical Treatment Act of 2009, H.R. 1549 and S. 619, which would prohibit the nontherapeutic feeding of medically important antibiotics to livestock. Addressing the House of Representatives last March, Representative Slaughter stressed the importance of the bill, urging that "unless we act now, we will unwittingly be permitting animals to serve as incubators for resistant bacteria."

Though opponents of the bill allege that a ban would increase meat costs to consumers, in reality consumers already pay the price for industry's reliance on antibiotics. In addition to being a major public health concern, antibiotic resistance increases healthcare costs by $4 to $5 billion a year.

Fortunately, through the use of responsible, humane management practices, farm animals can be raised under conditions which obviate the need for the prophylactic feeding of antibiotics. By increasing reliance on vaccinations, diligently monitoring animal health, and most importantly, by phasing out stressful confinement housing systems which compromise animals' immune systems and facilitate disease transmission, producers can manage animal diseases without resorting to the indiscriminate use of antibiotics.

AWI's own Animal Welfare Approved label prohibits the use of nontherapeutic antibiotics. Instead, farmers maintain herd health through vaccination, pasture management, exceptional hygiene, and the reduction of stressors which weaken animal immune systems. The Animal Welfare Approved program requires farmers to provide sick animals with appropriate medical treatment but promotes the use of antibiotics only for individual animals that need them, rather than as a means of compensating for unhealthy and inhumane living conditions.

Please write to your Representative and Senators asking them to cosponsor the Preservation of Antibiotics for Medical Treatment Act, H.R. 1549 and S. 619 and tell them that the nontherapeutic use of antibiotics on industrial farms jeopardizes human health while perpetuating a system of inhumane and irresponsible animal husbandry. The addresses can be found on the following page

Sheep Diseases

Sheep can be affected by a variety of infectious and noninfectious diseases. Some are contagious to people. These are called zoonotic diseases or zoonosis. Some diseases must be reported to government authorities. Certain diseases prevent the import and export of livestock.

Abomasal Emptying Defect (AED)

Abomasal emptying defect is a disease condition that has been observed mostly in Suffolk sheep over the age of two. For some unknown reason, the abomasum does not empty normally, causing it to enlarge. Affected sheep suffer a loss of appetite and weight. Although some animals may respond to treatment, the long term prognosis is usually poor. Until more is known about the disease, affected sheep and their offspring should not be kept for breeding.

Abortion

Abortion is when a ewe's pregnancy is terminated and she loses her lambs or she gives birth to weak or deformed lambs that die shortly after birth. There are both infectious and non-infectious causes of abortion. The most common infectious causes of abortion in ewes are *Chlamydia* (Enzootic abortion), *Campylobacter* (Vibrio), and *Toxoplasma gondii* (Toxoplasmosis). These organisms may also cause abortion (miscarriage) in women. As a precaution, pregnant women should not handle fetuses or placental fluids.

Brucellosis

Brucellosis is an infectious disease caused by bacteria of the genus *Brucella*. Various *Brucella* species affect sheep, goats, cattle, pigs, dogs, and other animals. In infected ruminants, brucellosis commonly causes abortion during the second half of gestation. Sheep are less susceptible than cattle, and brucellosis is not considered a common cause of abortion in sheep. Ovine brucellosis mainly affects rams, causing lesions in their reproductive organs.

Cache Valley Virus

Cache Valley Virus is an occasional cause of abortion outbreaks in sheep. It is spread by mosquitoes to pregnant ewes. If a ewe is infected at less than 28 days of gestation, the embryos usually die and are reabsorbed. If a ewe is infected after 45 days of pregnancy, there are usually no adverse effects.

If infection occurs between 28 and 45 days of gestation, the fetuses usually develop the "A-H syndrome," resulting in various congenital abnormalities affecting the central nervous system. Ewes that are infected usually show no signs of disease and develop a good immunity that lasts for several years. Cache Valley virus is similar to Akabanc Disease except that it only affects sheep.

Chlamydia

In the U.S., *Chlamydia* is the most common cause of abortion in ewes. It is transmitted from aborting sheep to other susceptible females. Ewe lambs are usually the most susceptible on farms where the organism is present. The bacteria which causes enzootic abortions in ewes is called *Chlamydia psittici*. *Chylamydia* causes abortion during the last month of pregnancy and may also result in the birth of lambs that die shortly after birth.

The organism may also cause pneumonia in young lambs, but the chlamydia species that causes abortion is not associated with conjunctivitis or arthritis. Chlamydia abortions can usually be stopped or reduced by treating the entire flock with tetracycline. A vaccine is available. It should be administered 60 days prior to breeding and repeated in 30 days, then annually just prior to breeding.

Leptospirosis

Sheep are generally more resistant to leptospirosis than cattle, swine, and most other domestic animals. Abortion due to this disease may occur during the last month of pregnancy. A blood test of aborting sheep will confirm diagnosis. The problem can be prevented with annual vaccination with a 5-strain leptospirosis vaccine.

Q Fever

Q Fever is a disease caused by the bacterium, *Coxiella burnetti*. The disease is found worldwide except for New Zealand. Sheep, goats, and cattle are most likely to get Q fever. The most common sign of Q fever is abortion during late pregnancy. However, most animals do not show any signs of illness. Animals get Q fever through contact with body fluids or secretions. Q fever is zoonotic (transmissble to people).

Rift Valley Fever

Rift valley disease is a viral disease of sub-Saharan Africa. The virus attacks the liver and causes symptoms ranging from fevers and listlessness to hemorrhage and abortion rates approaching 100% in pregnant sheep. It is transmitted by mosquitos. There is no specific therapy for infected animals.

Vaccination of animals against RVF has been used to prevent disease in endemic areas and to control epizootics. Rift Valley fever has not occurred in the United States. However, there has been concern that it could become permanently established in the U.S. if it does enter the country. Rift Valley fever is more deadly than West Nile virus.

Salmonella

In the U.S., salmonella abortion is a distant fourth in frequency as a cause of abortion in sheep, but probably occurs more often than recognised. The two major factors determining whether a pregnant ewe will abort from Salmonella are stress on the ewe and the number of Salmonella bacteria the ewe ingests.

Abortions may occur earlier in gestation, but are most common in the last month of gestation. Most of the ewes show diarrhea and some will die from metritis, peritonitis and septicemia. Healthy lambs may also contract the disease and die.

Toxoplasmosis

Toxoplasmosis is common cause of abortion in ewes. It is caused by *Toxoplasma gondii*, a protozoan parasite which causes coccidiosis in cats. Toxoplasma abortion in ewes follows ingestion of feed or water that has been contaminated with oocyte-laden cat feces. The organism migrates to the placenta and fetuses causing their death and expulsion. Ewes will abort during the last month of pregnancy or give birth to dead or weak lambs that usually die from starvation.

Infection in the first two months of gestation results in embryonic death and reabsorption. There is some evidence that Rumensin® and Deccox® will partially prevent toxoplasmosis in pregnant ewes. Limiting cat populations and preventing contamination of sheep feed and water with cat feces will help to prevent disease outbreaks. There is no vaccine available in the U.S. for toxoplasmosis.

Vibrio

Vibrio is the second most common cause of abortion in ewes. Abortion during the last month of pregnancy, stillborn lambs, and the birth of weak lambs are common signs of vibrio abortion The organisms which cause vibrio abortion are *Campylobacter jejuni* or *Campylobacter fetus*. Ewes are infected by oral ingestion. The incubation period from the time of infection and abortion is only two weeks. Vaccination can be effective in the face of an outbreak.

Acidosis

(lactic acidosis, ruminal acidois, grain overload, grain poisoning)

Lactic acidosis is caused by excess consumption of concentrates (grain) which results in high levels of acid being produced in the rumen. Affected sheep appear depressed and listless and may have abdominal pain. Acidosis can be a life-threatening condition. Affected sheep should be drenched with an antacid such as carmalax, bicarbonate of soda (baking soda), or products containing magnesium carbonate or magnesium hydroxide.

Acidosis can be prevented by proper feeding management. Concentrates (grain) should be introduced to the diet slowly and increased incrementally to give the rumen time to adjust.

Arthritis

Arthritis in sheep is an inflammation of the joints of the legs, resulting in loss of production, loss of carcass value and deaths. The main cause of arthritis in sheep is when bacteria enter the body via broken skin. The common times when a lamb will be susceptible to arthritis in this way are: 1) at or soon after birth with infection through the umbilical cord; 2) during docking, castration, and ear tagging; 3) through shearing wounds; and 4) other wounds.

There are several bacteria that may be implicated in arthritis. The most common is *Erysipelothix rhusiopathiae*. Signs appear 2 to 14 days after infection. Affected joints become swollen, hot, and painful, resulting in the lamb becoming reluctant to move. For most types of arthritis, the only treatment is a course of massive doses of antibiotics. Prevention is the result of good sanitation and hygiene.

Bacterial Meningitis

Bacterial meningitis occurs sporadically in lambs. It most commonly affects lambs 2 to 4 weeks old. The entry point of the bacteria is not clearly understood. Inadequate transfer of passive antibodies predisposes lambs to infection. Early clinical signs include depression, hunger, and failure to follow dams. Affected lambs may have abnormal gait. Their head is often held lower in a rigid extension. Response to treatment with antibiotics and corticosteroids is usually poor.

Bent Leg (a form of rickets)

Bent leg is a form of rickets and is due to a malfunction of bone metabolism during growth. It occurs during the rapid growth phase of the lamb, usually between 6 and 12 months of age. It occurs primarily in rams, but can occur in ewes. It is more common in Rambouillet and related breeds. Similar conditions occur in cattle, horses, dogs, poultry, and people.

It can be prevented by 1) feeding balanced rations; 2) avoiding the use of too much high energy or high protein feeds (rapid growth and nutritionally "pushing" animals for growth is a factor in all species for increased incidence of rickets); 3) providing a calcium to phosphorus ratio of at least 1.5 to 1; 4) supplementing the ration with 300 IU of vitamin D (per 100 lbs of body weight per day); 5) providing adequate magnesium; 6) shearing young rams in early winter to allow more skin surface for vitamin D conversion; and 7) providing housing that provides good exposure to sun during the winter.

Bloat

Bloat occurs when rumen gas production exceeds the rate of gas elimination. Gas then accumulates causing distention of the rumen. The skin on the left side of the animal behind the last rib may appear distended. Bloat can be a medical emergency, and timely intervention may be necessary to prevent death. Bloat is a common cause of sudden death in livestock. It usually results from nutritional causes.

There are two types of bloat: frothy and free gas.

Frothy Bloat (pasture bloat)

Frothy bloat is usually associated with the consumption of legumous forages, but may also occur in sheep grazing lush cereal grain pastures or wet grass pastures or consuming grain that is too finely ground. Animals with frothy bloat can be treated with anti-foaming agents such as cooking oil or mineral oil or a commercial product such as Poloxalene.

Free Gas Bloat (feed lot bloat)

Free grass bloat is associated with grain feeding and occurs when animals were not given enough of an adjustment period. Many of the same factors causing acidosis are associated with free-gas bloat. Simple passage of a stomach tube may be effective at relieving free gas bloat. Inserting a trochar or needle into the abdomen is a life-saving procedure that should only be attempted as a last resort.

Bluetongue

Bluetongue is an insect–transmitted, viral disease of sheep, cattle, goats, and other ruminants, such as white–tailed deer and pronghorn.

It is particularly damaging in sheep; half the sheep in an infected flock may die. In cattle and goats, however, bluetongue viruses cause very mild, self–limiting infections with only minor clinical consequences. A bluetongue virus infection causes inflammation, swelling, and hemorrhage of the mucous membranes of the mouth, nose, and tongue.

Inflammation and soreness of the feet also are associated with bluetongue. In sheep, the tongue and mucous membranes of the mouth become swollen, hemorrhagic, and may look red or dirty blue in colour, thus giving the disease its name. Bluetongue viruses are spread from animal to animal by biting gnats. In the United States, the disease is most prevalent in the southern and southwestern States.

Animals cannot directly contact the disease from other animals. The bluetongue vaccine for sheep is only effective against certain serotypes, will not prevent the disease, and may cause adverse reactions. Pregnant ewes should not be vaccinated.

Border Disease (hair-shaker disease, fuzzy lamb syndrome, BD)

Border disease is often seen in the newborn lamb which has a hairy coat and trembles uncontrollably. It is caused by a virus and causes a wide variety of symptoms depending upon the stage of pregnancy when the ewe becomes affected. Sheep affected by border disease are characterised by open ewes, abortion, weak and frail lambs, abnormal hair coat, and nervous symptoms that cause the lamb to shake.

The most common clinical symptom is abortion of macerated or mummified lambs. Border disease is usually brought into a flock by new additions that are carriers or when sheep are mixed with cattle that are shedding the Bovine viral disease virus. Bovine viral diarrhea vaccines for cattle cannot be recommended for use in sheep because border disease viruses most commonly isolated from sheep are antigenically distinct from bovine viral diarrhea viruses most common in cattle. There is no treatment and the disease will not respond to antibiotics.

Caseous Lymphadenitis (CLA, CL, boils, abscesses, cheesy gland)

Caseous lymphadenitis is an infectious, contagious disease that primarily affects the lymphatic system, though other organs can be affected. It is caused by the bacteria *Corynebacterium pseudotuberculosis*. Infection results in abscess formation in the lymph nodes which when cut or ruptured, discharge pus containing the bacteria into the immediate surroundings. When the nodes spread internally, affected ewes slowly lose weight and eventually become emaciated.

CL is the third leading cause of carcass condemnation in the U.S.. The disease is controlled by culling visible infected animals and practicing good hygiene at shearing time. There is a vaccine licensed for sheep. It has been shown to both decrease the number of abscesses in sheep and the number of sheep that develop abscesses.

Clostridial Diseases

Clostridial organisms of various types are found in the soil, where they can survive for a very long time. Most clostridial organisms can also occur quite naturally in the gut of healthy animals. Sheep can be infected with various clostridial diseases – black leg, botulism, malignant edema, red water disease, enterotoxemias (several types), and tetanus – but the most common are enterotoxemia types C & D and tetanus.

Enterotoxemia Type C (hemorrhagic enteritis, bloody scours)

Enterotoxemia type C is caused by *Clostridium perfringins* type C and affects lambs during their first few weeks of life, causing a bloody infection of the small intestine. It is often related to indigestion and predisposed by a sudden change in feed such as beginning creep feeding or sudden increase in milk supply. Treatment (antitoxin injected under the skin) is usually unrewarding Vaccination of pregnant ewes 30 days before lambing is recommended as prevention.

Enterotoxemia Type D ("classic" overeating disease, pulpy kidney disease)

Overeating disease is one of the most common sheep diseases in the world. It is caused by *Clostridium perfringins* type D and most commonly strikes the largest, fastest growing lambs in the flock. It is caused by a sudden change in feed that causes the organism, which is already present in the lamb's gut, to proliferate causing a toxic reaction. It is most commonly observed in lambs that are consuming high concentrate rations, but it can also occur when lambs are nursing heavy milking dams. It usually affects lambs over one month of age. Treatment (antitoxin injected under the skin) is usually unrewarding. Vaccination of pregnant ewes 30 days before lambing is recommended as prevention.

Tetanus (lock jaw)

Tetanus is caused by *Clostridium tetani*, a soil inhabitant that is a prolific spore producer. This disease is usually related to docking and castrating by elastrator bands, though any wound can harbor the tetanus organism.

Signs of tetanus occur from about four days to three weeks or longer after infection is established in a wound. The animal may have a stiff gait, "lockjaw" can develop and the third eyelid may protrude across the eye. The animal will usually go down with all four legs held out straight and stiff and the head drawn back. Convulsions may occur and the animal.

Treatment consists of the tetanus anti-serum and antibiotics. It is usually unrewarding. Tetanus can be prevented by vaccinating pregnant ewes 30 days before lambing. If pregnant ewes were not vaccinated for tetanus, the tetanus anti-toxin can be administered to lambs at the time of docking and/or castrating. The tetanus anti-toxin provides immediate short-term immunity and can be used at the time of docking and castrating to prevent disease outbreaks.

Grass Tetany (grass staggers, magnesium deficiency)

Grass tetany is a complex disease traditionally associated with a magnesium deficiency. All ruminants are susceptible. Magnesium deficiency in sheep most commonly occurs in acute form within 4-6 weeks of lambing. Affected ewes exhibit sensitivity to touch and trembling of the facial muscles; some are unable to move, others move stiffly; extreme cases collapse and show repeated tetanic spasms with all four limbs rigidly extended.

Low blood magnesium can be caused by low levels of magnesium in lush spring grass or by mineral imbalances such as high potassium and nitrogen or low calcium in the diet. Ewes with grass staggers are often low in calcium as well as magnesium. It is therefore wise to use a combined treatment of calcium borogluconate and magnesium hypophosphite. Producers can add about 10 to 20 grams of commercial or homemade supplemental magnesium to livestock diets to prevent grass tetany. Magnesium oxide is one of the best and cheapest magnesium sources.

Hypothermia (chilling)

Hypothermia is a leading cause of death in neonatal lambs. Mild to moderate hypothermia is characterised by a body temperature between 98° and 102°F. Severe hypothermia occurs when body temperature is below 98°F. Hypothermia is caused by excess body heat loss combined with reduced heat production. Newborn lambs are unable to regulate their body temperature during their first 36 hours.

Severely hypothermic lambs need to be removed from the ewe for treatment. If they are less than five hours old, they should receive an intraperitoneal injection of a warm 20 percent dextrose (glucose) solution. Wet lambs should be towel dried and supplemented with heat or put in a warming box using dry heat (heat lamp or hair drier). Colostrum should be tube fed at a rate of 20 to 25 ml per pound of body weight. Once rectal temperature is normal, lambs may be returned to their dams.

Losses due to hypothermia can be prevented by providing ewes with adequate shelter for lambing, shearing ewes prior to lambing, confining ewes and lambs for one or two days to promote bonding, checking ewes for adequate milk production, and helping lambs suckle to ensure adequate colostrum intake.

Internal Parasites

There are three broad types of internal parasite that can cause significant health issues in sheep: worms, flukes, and protozoa.

Cryptosporidiosis (Cryptosporidium sp.)

Cryptosporidium species are tiny protozoan parasites closely related to coccidia. One major species, *Cryptosporidium parvum*, infects both farm animals and humans. *C. parvum* has a rapid, direct life cycle and infection occurs when viable oocysts in the environment are ingested by susceptible hosts, usually lambs under a month old.

Lambs as young as 3 days can be affected. Lambs are depressed and reluctant to suck while the diarrhea lasts. Very young lambs soon become dehydrated and die. In poor weather conditions, lambs may die of hypothermia. The illness may last for up to 10 days, and relapses after apparent recovery are common.

Coccidiosis (Eimeria sp.)

Coccidia are single-cell protozoa that are naturally in the sheep's digestive system. Young lambs are particularly susceptible to coccidia especially during periods of stress (e.g. weaning). Coccidia damage the lining of the small intestine, affecting absorption of nutrients. The most common symptom of coccidiosis is diarrhea. The diarrhea may be bloody or smeared with mucous.

The diagnosis of coccidiosis cannot be confirmed by identification of oocysts in fecal samples. Coccidosis is mostly a management-related disease, caused by overstocking and poor hygiene. Coccidiosis can be prevented by including Lasolocid (Bovatec®), Monensin (Rumensin®), or Decoquinate (Deccox®) in the feed or mineral. Coccidiosis should be treated with Amprolium or sulfa medications.

Stomach Worms (Haemonchus, Trichostrongylus, and Ostertagia sp.)

The internal parasites of greatest concern in sheep are usually the stomach worms, with the barber pole worm (*Haemonchus Contortus*) being of primary concern and the small brown stomach worm being of secondary concern. The barber pole worm is a blood-sucking parasite that pierces the mucosa of the abomasum, causing blood and protein loss.

The primary symptom of barber pole infection is anemia (blood loss). Anemia can be observed in the sheep by examining its lower eyelid, which will become paler (whiter) with increasing infestation. An accumulation of fluid under the jaw, called "bottle jaw" is also a tell-tale of barber pole infection.

The small brown stomach worm also burrows into the lining of the abomasum, but it causes typical digestive symptoms, especially diarrhea. Microscopically, it is difficult to differentiate between the barber pole worm and the brown stomach worm. The eggs only differ in size not appearance.

Nematodirus Spp.

The life cycle and transmission of Nematodirus differs from that of other sheep worms. Infective *N. battus* larvae generally don't survive for long on pasture when weather conditions are warm and dry, but can survive for several months during cool and damp weather. The symptoms of nematodirus are scours, weight loss, and sudden death.

Tapeworms (Moniezia sp.)

There is disagreement as to whether tapeworms cause serious problems in sheep. They are generally considered to be non-pathogenic, though they can cause weight loss, diarrhea, and even death in extreme cases. The only anthelmintics that are effective against tapeworms are the benzamidizoles (fenbendazole and albendazole). Most research shows no benefit to treating lambs for tapeworms. Tapeworms are the only parasite that is visible in the feces.

Lungworms

Lungworm larvae are passed in the feces, but travel to the respiratory system once they enter the sheep system. The symptoms of lung worm infection are not obvious unless the problem is severe.

Lungworm infestations are most commonly diagnosed at necropsy or slaughter. The same anthelmintics that are effective against stomach worms are also effective against lung worms.

Liver Flukes (Fasciola hepatica)

Liver flukes can be problematic in wet areas. They are spread by snails and slugs. As the name would suggest, liver flukes damage the liver of the host animal. They cause blood loss, diarrhea, weight loss, and death. The only drugs that are effective against liver flukes (the adult form) are clorsulon (contained in Ivomec® Plus) and albendazole (Valbazan®).

Meningeal Worm (Paralaphostrongylus tenius, deer worm, brain worm)

The meningeal worm is a parasite of the White Tail deer. Sheep, goats, llamas, alpacas, and horses are abnormal hosts for the parasite. After they ingest the larvae, the larvae travel to the spinal cord causing gait abnormalities and eventually paralysis. When the parasite reaches the sheep's brain, it will kill them.

Meningeal worm infection cannot be detected in the live animal. When meningeal worm is suspected, high doses of anthelmintics and anti-inflammatory drugs are recommended. Infections can be prevented by limiting exposure to deer or by controlling snail populations, since the parasite requires snails to complete its life cycle.

Johne's Disease (paratuberculosis)

Johne's Disease (pronounced "Yo nees") is a disease that affects the intestines of mostly ruminants. It is most commonly observed in dairy cows, but may also affect beef cattle, sheep, and goats. It is caused by a hardy bacteria called *Mycobacterium paratuberculosis*. The strain that affects sheep is different than the one that affects cows, though there is an intermediate strain that sheep are susceptible to. While cattle experience diarrhea, in sheep, Johne's tends to be more of a wasting disease. Control of the disease in infected flocks is difficult due to the lack of a reliable live animal test. Vaccination will reduce the number of clinical cases in a flock, but will not prevent all animals from becoming infected. Colostrum from other sources (cows, goats) could be a source of infection in sheep flocks. The is no treatment for Johne's disease.

Joint or Navel Ill

Joint ill occurs in lambs up to one month of age. Affected lambs are often lame in several joints, usually limb joints, including fetlocks, knees, hocks and stifles. Affected joints are hot and painful. The lambs are dull, feverish and clearly unthrifty. Some may have swollen, infected navels, while others may have symptoms of pneumonia or meningitis.

The infection is usually caused by strains of *streptococci*, though coliforms and occasionally *Actinomyces pyogenes* may be isolated. Affected lambs should be treated with a long-acting penicillin. Joint ill is prevented by good hygiene and using a navel dip, such as betadine or gentle iodine.

Lameness

It has been estimated that 80 percent of the flocks in Great Britain have lame sheep. Lameness can be a sign of several foot conditions – some of which are very serious – as well as some other problems. These include foot rot and scald, strawberry foot, foot abscess, foot-and-mouth disease, bluetongue, ovine interdigital dermatitis (looks like scald), sore mouth, arthritis, nutritional deficiencies, mineral excesses, and physical injuries. The more common foot problems can be avoided or minimised if good husbandry practices are followed. Regular hoof inspection and foot paring will prevent many problems.

Laminitis (founder)

Lameness related to laminitis is caused by an inadequate flow of blood in the foot. Signs are heat in the feet. Laminitis is normally associated with digestive problems resulting from excessive intake of grain (grain overload/acidosis), which usually masks the effects on the feet. Such animals usually die before the feet become involved. Recovered animals may exhibit foot growth and/or permanent lameness. Feeding management is key to the prevention of laminitis/founder.

Listeriosis (circling disease)

Listeria monocytogenes, the bacteria that causes listeriosis, is widely distributed in nature and is found in soil, feedstuffs, and feces from healthy animals. It is most commonly associated with the feeding of moldy silage or spoiled hay, but because the organism lives naturally in the environment, listeriosis may occur sporadically.

Listeriosis usually presents itself as encephalitis (inflammation of the brain), but may also cause abortion in ewes. Sheep with the neurological form of the disease become depressed and disoriented. They may walk in circles with a head tilt and facial paralysis. Mortality is high and treatment (high doses of antibiotics) is generally not effective.

Mastitis (hard bag, blue bag)

Mastitis is an inflammation of the mammary gland (udder) which is usually caused by a bacterial infection. The bacteria causing mastitis in ewes are *Staphylococcus aureus* and *Pasteurella hemolytica*. There are two types of mastitis: acute and chronic. The glands of ewes with acute mastitis may be discoloured and dark, swollen and very warm. The affected ewe may be reluctant to walk, may hold up one rear foot, and may not permit her lambs to nurse.

Ewes with chronic mastitis often go undetected. Mastitis is usually treated with intramammary infusions of antibiotics and systemic antibiotics. There is no vaccine for mastitis. It is best prevented by good management and sanitation.

Measles (sheep measles, cysticerosis)

Sheep measles (*Cysticercus ovis*) is the intermediate or larval stage of the cestode (tapeworm) Taenia ovis, the adult stage of which is found in the small intestine of dogs (sheep host the larvae stage). Sheep measle lesions are found in the heart, diaphragm and other muscles of sheep and goats. Although not considered to be a human health hazard, carcasses can be condemned on account of sheep measles.

There are no clinical signs of cysticerosis in sheep. Currently diagnosis is only made by finding the cysts at slaughter. To prevent sheep measles, dogs and other canines should not be allowed to feed on sheep or goat carcasses. Dogs should be dewormed for tapeworms. Any dog given access to the farm should be required to be dewormed.

Milk Fever (hypocalcemia, parturient paresis)

Milk fever is a metabolic disease affecting mostly pregnant ewes near term when calcium requirements are the highest. It is most commonly caused by an inadequate intake of calcium, but can also be caused by a ewe's inability to mobilise calcium reserves prior to or after lambing. Milk fever presents similar symptoms as pregnancy toxemia but can be differentiated by the affected ewe's response to calcium therapy.

Ewes in the early stages of milk fever can be administered calcium gluconate subcutaneously. More seriously affected ewes will require intravenous calcium and other supportive therapies. Milk fever can be prevented by providing proper levels of calcium in ewe diets, especially during late gestation.

Ovine Progressive Pneumonia (OPP, lunger disease. Maedi-Visna)

Ovine progressive pneumonia is a slow developing viral disease that is characterised by progressive weight loss, difficulty in breathing and development of lameness, paralysis, and mastitis. It is very closely related to caprine arthritis-encephalitis virus (CAE) and is caused by a retrovirus. The OPP virus closely resembles Maedi-Visna which is a similar slow or retrovirus found in other parts of the world.

OPP is transmitted laterally to other susceptible animals or to offspring through ingestion of infected milk and colostrum. Veterinary diagnostic laboratory assistance is required for diagnosis. There is no treatment, but OPP can be eliminated from the herd using annual blood testing and removal of positive animals and removal of the lambs from the ewes prior to suckling.

It is estimated that over 50% of the flocks in the U.S. are infected with OPP with the number of sheep infected within a positive flock anywhere between 1% to 70%. However, the vast majority of infected sheep will never show respiratory disease or a wasting syndrome.

Pink Eye (infectious keratoconjunctivitis)

Pinkeye is a highly contagious disease affecting the eyes of sheep. Pinkeye may result from many different infective agents: Chlamydia, certain viruses, and mycoplasma. The disease will usually complete its course in three weeks in individual sheep. The use of eye medications containing antibiotics may be helpful in individual cases. There are no effective vaccines available, as the agent that causes pinkeye in sheep and goats is different from the one that causes it in cattle.

Pizzle Rot (sheath rot)

Pizzle rot is an infection in the sheath area of the ram. It is caused by the bacteria, *Corynebacterium renale* or one from that group. The other factor is high protein diets (>16 percent). Ammonia, produced by the excess urea in the ram's urine can cause severe irritation and ulceration of the skin around the preputial opening. The debris from the ulcer form a crust which may block the opening to the prepuce. Pizzle rot can affect a ram's desire and ability to mate.

Plant Poisoning

It is important to consider plant toxicities when diagnosing death losses. Many plants are toxic or potentially toxic to sheep. Some plants accumulate toxins during specific times of their growing cycle or after periods of environmental stress. The incidence of plant poisoning in livestock tends to increase when normal forages are scarce, causing animals to eat plants that they would not normally eat. The signs of plant poisoning are as varied as the plants themselves and may mimic other diseases.

Many poisonous plants cause sudden death. Some plants cause photosensitisation (a severe skin reaction). Other poisonous plants affect the nervous system. Some plant poisonings can be treated, if signs are recognised early. For many plant toxins, there are no treatments.

Pneumonia (respiratory disease complex, pasteurellosis, shipping fever)

Pneumonia is second in importance to diseases of the digestive tract. Pneumonia is a respiratory complex with no single agent being solely responsible for the disease. The most common bacteria isolated from respiratory infections is *Pasteurella haemolytica* or *Pasteurella multocida* or both. Affected animals become depressed and go off feed.

They may cough and show some respiratory distress. Temperatures are usually over 104°F. The disease may be acute with sudden deaths or take a course of several days. Pneumonia is treated with antibiotics.

Polioencephalomalacia (PEM, CCN, polio, cerebrocortical necrosis)

Polioencephalomalacia is a disease of the central nervous system, caused by a vitamin B1 (thiamine) deficiency. Since the rumen manufactures B vitamins, polio is not caused by insufficient thiamine, but rather the inability to utilise it.

The most common symptom of polio is blindness and star-gazing. Polio most commonly occurs in lambs that are consuming high concentrate diets. Polio can also occur in sheep that consume plants that contain a thiamase inhibitor. Polio symptoms mimic other neurological disease conditions, but a differential diagnosis can be made based on the animals' response to injections of vitamin B1.

Polyarthritis

Polyarthritis is an infectious disease of nursing lambs, recently weaned lambs, and feedlot lambs. Symptoms are stiffness, reluctance to move, depression, loss of body weight, and conjunctivitis. Clinically the disease is primarily characterised by stiffness and by conjunctivitis. Body temperatures over 104°F are common. Lambs can be treated with several different broad-spectrum antibiotics or tetracycline drugs.

Pregnancy Toxemia (ketosis, twin lamb disease, lambing paralysis, hypoglycemia)

Pregnancy toxemia is a metabolic disease that affects ewes during late gestation. It most commonly afflicts thin ewes, overfat ewes, older ewes, and/or ewes carrying multiple fetuses. It is caused by an inadequate intake of energy during late pregnancy, when the majority of fetal growth is occurring.

Treatment is to increase the blood sugar supply to the body by administering glucose intravenously or propylene glycol or molasses orally. In extreme cases, removal of the fetuses is the only recourse to save the ewe and lambs.

Pregnancy toxemia can be prevented by providing adequate energy to ewes during late gestation, usually ½ to 1 lb. of grain per head per day, more for high producing ewes. Adequate feeder space is also necessary to ensure all ewes are able to consume enough feed.

Rabies

Rabies is a viral disease of the central nervous system of mammals, spread by contact with saliva from an infected animal, usually through bites or scratches, abrasions, or open wounds in the skin. Domestic animals may become exposed during normal grazing or roaming. Sheep have symptoms similar to cattle, and sometimes vigourously pull their wool. Livestock and horse owners may decide to vaccinate their animals if they are often exposed to potentially rabid wild or domestic animals.

Generally, production animals, such as dairy cow herds and sheep flocks, are not vaccinated because the potential risks are usually lower than the annual costs of vaccination and because human contact with individual animals is low. Small groups of valuable purebred animals may be an exception. In recent years, a few states have required vaccination for rabies before an animal (including some livestock) can be exhibited publicly.

Rectal Prolapse

A rectal prolpase is protrusion of the rectal tissue through the exterior of the body. It usually begins as a small round area that sticks out when the lamb lays down or coughs. In extreme cases, the intestines can pass through the opening and the disease can be fatal. There are many predisposing factors to rectal prolapses, including genetics, short tail docks, coughing, weather, stress, and high concentrate diets.

Rectal prolapses tend to occur more in ewe lambs than wether lambs and more in black-faced sheep than white-faced sheep. The link between extreme tail docking and the incidence of rectal prolapses in grain-fed lambs has been scientifically established. Usually, lambs with prolapsed rectums are prematurely slaughtered or sent to market. It is possible to repair a rectal prolapse by amputating the prolapsed part of the rectum. These lambs should not be kept for breeding.

Ringwomb

Ringwomb is when the cervix fails to dilate sufficiently to allow delivery of the lamb(s). While sometimes the cervix of affected ewes can be opened with gentle pressure or the injection of hormones, usually such efforts prove futile and a caesarian section to remove the lambs is the only option that will produce a successful outcome. Unfortunately, little is known about the cause of ringworm and how to prevent it. There is some evidence to suggest that ringwomb has a genetic link.

Ringworm (club lamb fungus, wool rot, and lumpy wool)

Club lamb fungus is a highly contagious fungal infection of the skin of sheep. It is primarily a problem with show lambs that are frequently slick sheared. Club Lamb Fungus is caused by fungus of the genus *Trichophyton*. Infection occurs when the fungus invades the skin and hair (wool) follicles. Fungal spores are transmitted by contaminated clippers, blankets, combs, bedding, bunks, and pens. Lesions can appear anywhere, however, most are found on the head, neck, and back. The infection is susceptible to anti-fungal agents. Club lamb fungus causes a nasty ringworm infection in people.

Ryegrass Staggers

Ryegrass staggers is a disease of grazing animals that causes muscle spasms, loss of muscle control and paralysis. It is caused by a group of toxins that accumulates in the leaf sheaths of perennial ryegrass. The toxins are produced by a native fungus called ryegrass endophyte, *Neotyphodium lolii*, that grows within the leaves, stems and seeds of perennial ryegrass. Sheep and cattle are most commonly affected but horses, aplaca and deer are also susceptible.

Ryegrass staggers has not been recorded in goats. Affected animals have a stiff gait or are unable to walk. They may injure or kill themselves in transit. The toxins can induce high body temperatures thus animals will try to cool themselves. Younger animals tend to be worst affected. The symptoms of ryegrass staggers usually develop 7-

14 days after livestock stock start grazing the toxic parts of the plant. Prolonged exposure to toxic pasture can lead to permanent neurological damage.

Scrapie

Scrapie is a fatal disease affecting the central nervous system of sheep and goats. It is spread from the dam to her offspring and other lambs (and kids) that come into contact with her birthing fluids, placenta, and bedding soiled with birthing fluids. There is not treatment for scrapie. Affected animals always die.

While the occurrence of scrapie in the U.S. sheep flock is low, it is a disease of regulatory concern. This is because scrapie is a member of a family of diseases called "transmissible spongiform encephalopathies (TGE's), which also includes chronic wasting disease (in mule deer and elk), mad cow disease (bovine spongiform encephalopathy) and classic and new variant Creutzfeldt-Jacob's Disease (in humans).

Producers of breeding stock are encouraged to enrolled in the voluntary scrapie flock certification program, which after five years of scrapie-free monitoring, enables a flock to be certified "scrapie-free." Furthermore, while scrapie is not a genetic disease, a sheep's genetic make-up influences its susceptibility to scrapie if exposed to the infective agent. Therefore, sheep can be tested for scrapie resistance.

Scrotal Hernia

A scrotal hernia is when the ram's intestines slip through the inguinal rings into the scrotum. The condition causes an enlargement of the scrotum. Scrotal hernias may be congenital or acquired. They are thought to be caused by trauma. It is not known if genetics plays a role. While it may be possible to surgically repair a scrotal hernia, a more practical option would be harvest them for meat. Obviously, rams with scrotal hernias should not be used for breeding.

Soremouth (contagious ecthyma, scabby mouth, pustular dermatitis, orf)

Soremouth is the most common skin disease affecting sheep (and goats). It is a highly contagious viral infection that can also produce painful human infections. The virus causes scab formation on the skin, usually around the mouth, nostrils, eyes, mammary gland and vulva. It first appears as tiny red nodules, usually at the junction of the lips. Treatment is usually unrewarding. The disease will usually run its course in 1 to 4 weeks.

Effective vaccines are available. The vaccine is applied to a woolless area in the inside of the ear or under a leg where it cannot spread to the mouths of other animals. Once the vaccine is used on the premises, it should be continued yearly. Flocks that have not experienced soremouth should probably not vaccinate for soremouth, since the vaccine introduces the virus to the farm.

Grass Tetany (grass staggers, magnesium deficiency)

Grass tetany is a complex disease traditionally associated with a magnesium deficiency. All ruminants are susceptible. Magnesium deficiency in sheep most commonly occurs in acute form within 4-6 weeks of lambing. Affected ewes exhibit sensitivity to touch and trembling of the facial muscles; some are unable to move, others move stiffly; extreme cases collapse and show repeated tetanic spasms with all four limbs rigidly extended.

Low blood magnesium can be caused by low levels of magnesium in lush spring grass or by mineral imbalances such as high potassium and nitrogen or low calcium in the diet. Ewes with grass staggers are often low in calcium as well as magnesium. It is therefore wise to use a combined treatment of calcium borogluconate and magnesium hypophosphite. Producers can add about 10 to 20 grams of commercial or homemade supplemental magnesium to livestock diets to prevent grass tetany. Magnesium oxide is one of the best and cheapest magnesium sources.

Hypothermia (chilling)

Hypothermia is a leading cause of death in neonatal lambs. Mild to moderate hypothermia is characterised by a body temperature between 98° and 102°F. Severe hypothermia occurs when body temperature is below 98°F.

Hypothermia is caused by excess body heat loss combined with reduced heat production. Newborn lambs are unable to regulate their body temperature during their first 36 hours.

Severely hypothermic lambs need to be removed from the ewe for treatment. If they are less than five hours old, they should receive an intraperitoneal injection of a warm 20 percent dextrose (glucose) solution. Wet lambs should be towel dried and supplemented with heat or put in a warming box using dry heat (heat lamp or hair drier). Colostrum should be tube fed at a rate of 20 to 25 ml per pound of body weight. Once rectal temperature is normal, lambs may be returned to their dams.

Losses due to hypothermia can be prevented by providing ewes with adequate shelter for lambing, shearing ewes prior to lambing, confining ewes and lambs for one or two days to promote bonding, checking ewes for adequate milk production, and helping lambs suckle to ensure adequate colostrum intake.

Internal Parasites

There are three broad types of internal parasite that can cause significant health issues in sheep: worms, flukes, and protozoa.

Cryptosporidiosis (Cryptosporidium sp.)

Cryptosporidium species are tiny protozoan parasites closely related to coccidia. One major species, *Cryptosporidium parvum*, infects both farm animals and humans. *C. parvum* has a rapid, direct life cycle and infection occurs when viable oocysts in the environment are ingested by susceptible hosts, usually lambs under a month old.

Lambs as young as 3 days can be affected. Lambs are depressed and reluctant to suck while the diarrhea lasts. Very young lambs soon become dehydrated and die. In poor weather conditions, lambs may die of hypothermia. The illness may last for up to 10 days, and relapses after apparent recovery are common.

Coccidiosis (Eimeria sp.)

Coccidia are single-cell protozoa that are naturally in the sheep's digestive system. Young lambs are particularly susceptible to coccidia especially during periods of stress (e.g. weaning). Coccidia damage the lining of the small intestine, affecting absorption of nutrients. The most common symptom of coccidiosis is diarrhea. The diarrhea may be bloody or smeared with mucous.

The diagnosis of coccidiosis cannot be confirmed by identification of oocysts in fecal samples. Coccidosis is mostly a management-related disease, caused by overstocking and poor hygiene. Coccidiosis can be prevented by including Lasolocid (Bovatec®), Monensin (Rumensin®), or Decoquinate (Deccox®) in the feed or mineral. Coccidiosis should be treated with Amprolium or sulfa medications.

Stomach Worms (Haemonchus, Trichostrongylus, and Ostertagia sp.)

The internal parasites of greatest concern in sheep are usually the stomach worms, with the barber pole worm (*Haemonchus Contortus*) being of primary concern and the small brown stomach worm being of secondary concern. The barber pole worm is a blood-sucking parasite that pierces the mucosa of the abomasum, causing blood and protein loss.

The primary symptom of barber pole infection is anemia (blood loss). Anemia can be observed in the sheep by examining its lower eyelid, which will become paler (whiter) with increasing infestation. An accumulation of fluid under the jaw, called "bottle jaw" is also a tell-tale of barber pole infection.

The small brown stomach worm also burrows into the lining of the abomasum, but it causes typical digestive symptoms, especially diarrhea. Microscopically, it is difficult to differentiate between the barber pole worm and the brown stomach worm. The eggs only differ in size not appearance.

Nematodirus Spp.

The life cycle and transmission of Nematodirus differs from that of other sheep worms. Infective *N. battus* larvae generally don't survive for long on pasture when weather conditions are warm and dry, but can survive for several months during cool and damp weather. The symptoms of nematodirus are scours, weight loss, and sudden death.

Tapeworms (Moniezia sp.)

There is disagreement as to whether tapeworms cause serious problems in sheep. They are generally considered to be non-pathogenic, though they can cause weight loss, diarrhea, and even death in extreme cases. The only anthelmintics that are effective against tapeworms are the benzamidizoles (fenbendazole and albendazole). Most research shows no benefit to treating lambs for tapeworms. Tapeworms arc the only parasite that is visible in the feces.

Lungworms

Lungworm larvae are passed in the feces, but travel to the respiratory system once they enter the sheep system. The symptoms of lung worm infection are not obvious unless the problem is severe. Lungworm infestations are most commonly diagnosed at necropsy or slaughter. The same anthelmintics that are effective against stomach worms are also effective against lung worms.

Liver Flukes (Fasciola hepatica)

Liver flukes can be problematic in wet areas. They are spread by snails and slugs. As the name would suggest, liver flukes damage the liver of the host animal. They cause blood loss, diarrhea, weight loss, and death. The only drugs that are effective against liver flukes (the adult form) are clorsulon (contained in Ivomec® Plus) and albendazole (Valbazan®).

Meningeal Worm (Paralaphostrongylus tenius, deer worm, brain worm)

The meningeal worm is a parasite of the White Tail deer. Sheep, goats, llamas, alpacas, and horses are abnormal hosts for the parasite. After they ingest the larvae, the larvae travel to the spinal cord causing gait abnormalities and eventually paralysis. When the parasite reaches the sheep's brain, it will kill them.

Meningeal worm infection cannot be detected in the live animal. When meningeal worm is suspected, high doses of anthelmintics and anti-inflammatory drugs are recommended. Infections can be prevented by limiting exposure to deer or by controlling snail populations, since the parasite requires snails to complete its life cycle.

Johne's Disease (paratuberculosis)

Johne's Disease (pronounced "Yo nees") is a disease that affects the intestines of mostly ruminants. It is most commonly observed in dairy cows, but may also affect beef cattle, sheep, and goats. It is caused by a hardy bacteria called *Mycobacterium paratuberculosis*. The strain that affects sheep is different than the one that affects cows, though there is an intermediate strain that sheep are susceptible to.

While cattle experience diarrhea, in sheep, Johne's tends to be more of a wasting disease. Control of the disease in infected flocks is difficult due to the lack of a reliable live animal test. Vaccination will reduce the number of clinical cases in a flock, but will not prevent all animals from becoming infected. Colostrum from other sources (cows, goats) could be a source of infection in sheep flocks. The is no treatment for Johne's disease.

Joint or Navel Ill

Joint ill occurs in lambs up to one month of age. Affected lambs are often lame in several joints, usually limb joints, including fetlocks, knees, hocks and stifles. Affected joints are hot and painful. The lambs are dull, feverish and clearly unthrifty. Some may have swollen, infected navels, while others may have symptoms of pneumonia or meningitis.

The infection is usually caused by strains of *streptococci*, though coliforms and occasionally *Actinomyces pyogenes* may be isolated. Affected lambs should be treated with a long-acting penicillin. Joint ill is prevented by good hygiene and using a navel dip, such as betadine or gentle iodine.

Lameness

It has been estimated that 80 percent of the flocks in Great Britain have lame sheep. Lameness can be a sign of several foot conditions – some of which are very serious – as well as some other problems. These include foot rot and scald, strawberry foot, foot abscess, foot-and-mouth disease, bluetongue, ovine interdigital dermatitis (looks like scald), sore mouth, arthritis, nutritional deficiencies, mineral excesses, and physical injuries. The more common foot problems can be avoided or minimised if good husbandry practices are followed. Regular hoof inspection and foot paring will prevent many problems.

Laminitis (founder)

Lameness related to laminitis is caused by an inadequate flow of blood in the foot. Signs are heat in the feet. Laminitis is normally associated with digestive problems resulting from excessive intake of grain (grain overload/acidosis), which usually masks the effects on the feet. Such animals usually die before the feet become involved. Recovered animals may exhibit foot growth and/or permanent lameness. Feeding management is key to the prevention of laminitis/founder.

Listeriosis (circling disease)

Listeria monocytogenes, the bacteria that causes listeriosis, is widely distributed in nature and is found in soil, feedstuffs, and feces from healthy animals. It is most commonly associated with the feeding of moldy silage or spoiled hay, but because the organism lives naturally in the environment, listeriosis may occur sporadically.

Listeriosis usually presents itself as encephalitis (inflammation of the brain), but may also cause abortion in ewes. Sheep with the neurological form of the disease become depressed and disoriented. They may walk in circles with a head tilt and facial paralysis. Mortality is high and treatment (high doses of antibiotics) is generally not effective.

Mastitis (hard bag, blue bag)

Mastitis is an inflammation of the mammary gland (udder) which is usually caused by a bacterial infection. The bacteria causing mastitis in ewes are *Staphylococcus aureus* and *Pasteurella hemolytica*. There are two types of mastitis: acute and chronic. The glands of ewes with acute mastitis may be discoloured and dark, swollen and very warm. The affected ewe may be reluctant to walk, may hold up one rear foot, and may not permit her lambs to nurse.

Ewes with chronic mastitis often go undetected. Mastitis is usually treated with intramammary infusions of antibiotics and systemic antibiotics. There is no vaccine for mastitis. It is best prevented by good management and sanitation.

Measles (sheep measles, cysticerosis)

Sheep measles (*Cysticercus ovis*) is the intermediate or larval stage of the cestode (tapeworm) Taenia ovis, the adult stage of which is found in the small intestine of dogs (sheep host the larvae stage). Sheep measle lesions are found in the heart, diaphragm and other muscles of sheep and goats. Although not considered to be a human health hazard, carcasses can be condemned on account of sheep measles.

There are no clinical signs of cysticerosis in sheep. Currently diagnosis is only made by finding the cysts at slaughter. To prevent sheep measles, dogs and other canines should not be allowed to feed on sheep or goat carcasses. Dogs should be dewormed for tapeworms. Any dog given access to the farm should be required to be dewormed.

Milk Fever (hypocalcemia, parturient paresis)

Milk fever is a metabolic disease affecting mostly pregnant ewes near term when calcium requirements are the highest. It is most commonly caused by an inadequate intake of calcium, but can also be caused by a ewe's inability to mobilise calcium reserves prior to or after lambing. Milk fever presents similar symptoms as pregnancy toxemia but can be differentiated by the affected ewe's response to calcium therapy.

Ewes in the early stages of milk fever can be administered calcium gluconate subcutaneously. More seriously affected ewes will require intravenous calcium and other supportive therapies. Milk fever can be prevented by providing proper levels of calcium in ewe diets, especially during late gestation.

Ovine Progressive Pneumonia (OPP, lunger disease. Maedi-Visna)

Ovine progressive pneumonia is a slow developing viral disease that is characterised by progressive weight loss, difficulty in breathing and development of lameness, paralysis, and mastitis. It is very closely related to caprine arthritis-encephalitis virus (CAE) and is caused by a retrovirus. The OPP virus closely resembles Maedi-Visna which is a similar slow or retrovirus found in other parts of the world.

OPP is transmitted laterally to other susceptible animals or to offspring through ingestion of infected milk and colostrum. Veterinary diagnostic laboratory assistance is required for diagnosis. There is no treatment, but OPP can be eliminated from the herd using annual blood testing and removal of positive animals and removal of the lambs from the ewes prior to suckling.

It is estimated that over 50% of the flocks in the U.S. are infected with OPP with the number of sheep infected within a positive flock anywhere between 1% to 70%. However, the vast majority of infected sheep will never show respiratory disease or a wasting syndrome.

Pink Eye (infectious keratoconjunctivitis)

Pinkeye is a highly contagious disease affecting the eyes of sheep. Pinkeye may result from many different infective agents: Chlamydia, certain viruses, and mycoplasma. The disease will usually complete its course in three weeks in individual sheep. The use of eye medications containing antibiotics may be helpful in individual cases. There are no effective vaccines available, as the agent that causes pinkeye in sheep and goats is different from the one that causes it in cattle.

Pizzle Rot (sheath rot)

Pizzle rot is an infection in the sheath area of the ram. It is caused by the bacteria, *Corynebacterium renale* or one from that group. The other factor is high protein diets (>16 percent). Ammonia, produced by the excess urea in the ram's urine can cause severe irritation and ulceration of the skin around the preputial opening. The debris from the ulcer form a crust which may block the opening to the prepuce. Pizzle rot can affect a ram's desire and ability to mate.

Plant Poisoning

It is important to consider plant toxicities when diagnosing death losses. Many plants are toxic or potentially toxic to sheep. Some plants accumulate toxins during specific times of their growing cycle or after periods of environmental stress. The incidence of plant poisoning in livestock tends to increase when normal forages are scarce, causing animals to eat plants that they would not normally eat.

The signs of plant poisoning are as varied as the plants themselves and may mimic other diseases. Many poisonous plants cause sudden death. Some plants cause photosensitisation (a severe skin reaction). Other poisonous plants affect the nervous system. Some plant poisonings can be treated, if signs are recognised early. For many plant toxins, there are no treatments.

Pneumonia (respiratory disease complex, pasteurellosis, shipping fever)

Pneumonia is second in importance to diseases of the digestive tract. Pneumonia is a respiratory complex with no single agent being solely responsible for the disease. The most common bacteria isolated from respiratory infections is *Pasteurella haemolytica* or *Pasteurella multocida* or both. Affected animals become depressed and go off feed. They may cough and show some respiratory distress. Temperatures are usually over 104°F. The disease may be acute with sudden deaths or take a course of several days. Pneumonia is treated with antibiotics.

Polioencephalomalacia (PEM, CCN, polio, cerebrocortical necrosis)

Polioencephalomalacia is a disease of the central nervous system, caused by a vitamin B1 (thiamine) deficiency. Since the rumen manufactures B vitamins, polio is not caused by insufficient thiamine, but rather the inability to utilise it. The most common symptom of polio is blindness and star-gazing.

Polio most commonly occurs in lambs that are consuming high concentrate diets. Polio can also occur in sheep that consume plants that contain a thiamase inhibitor. Polio symptoms mimic other neurological disease conditions, but a differential diagnosis can be made based on the animals' response to injections of vitamin B1.

Polyarthritis

Polyarthritis is an infectious disease of nursing lambs, recently weaned lambs, and feedlot lambs. Symptoms are stiffness, reluctance to move, depression, loss of body weight, and conjunctivitis. Clinically the disease is primarily characterised by stiffness and by conjunctivitis. Body temperatures over 104°F are common. Lambs can be treated with several different broad-spectrum antibiotics or tetracycline drugs.

Pregnancy Toxemia (ketosis, twin lamb disease, lambing paralysis, hypoglycemia)

Pregnancy toxemia is a metabolic disease that affects ewes during late gestation. It most commonly afflicts thin ewes, overfat ewes, older ewes, and/or ewes carrying multiple fetuses. It is caused by an inadequate intake of energy during late pregnancy, when the majority of fetal growth is occurring.

Treatment is to increase the blood sugar supply to the body by administering glucose intravenously or propylene glycol or molasses orally. In extreme cases, removal of the fetuses is the only recourse to save the ewe and lambs.

Pregnancy toxemia can be prevented by providing adequate energy to ewes during late gestation, usually ½ to 1 lb. of grain per head per day, more for high producing ewes. Adequate feeder space is also necessary to ensure all ewes are able to consume enough feed.

Rabies

Rabies is a viral disease of the central nervous system of mammals, spread by contact with saliva from an infected animal, usually through bites or scratches, abrasions, or open wounds in the skin. Domestic animals may become exposed during normal grazing or roaming. Sheep have symptoms similar to cattle, and sometimes vigourously pull their wool. Livestock and horse owners may decide to vaccinate their animals if they are often exposed to potentially rabid wild or domestic animals.

Generally, production animals, such as dairy cow herds and sheep flocks, are not vaccinated because the potential risks are usually lower than the annual costs of vaccination and because human contact with individual animals is low. Small groups of valuable purebred animals may be an exception. In recent years, a few states have required vaccination for rabies before an animal (including some livestock) can be exhibited publicly.

Rectal Prolapse

A rectal prolpase is protrusion of the rectal tissue through the exterior of the body. It usually begins as a small round area that sticks out when the lamb lays down or coughs. In extreme cases, the intestines can pass through the opening and the disease can be fatal. There are many predisposing factors to rectal prolapses, including genetics, short tail docks, coughing, weather, stress, and high concentrate diets.

Rectal prolapses tend to occur more in ewe lambs than wether lambs and more in black-faced sheep than white-faced sheep. The link between extreme tail docking and the incidence of rectal prolapses in grain-fed lambs has been scientifically established. Usually, lambs with prolapsed rectums are prematurely slaughtered or sent to market. It is possible to repair a rectal prolapse by amputating the prolapsed part of the rectum. These lambs should not be kept for breeding.

Ringwomb

Ringwomb is when the cervix fails to dilate sufficiently to allow delivery of the lamb(s). While sometimes the cervix of affected ewes can be opened with gentle pressure or the injection of hormones, usually such efforts prove futile and a caesarian section to remove the lambs is the only option that will produce a successful outcome. Unfortunately, little is known about the cause of ringworm and how to prevent it. There is some evidence to suggest that ringwomb has a genetic link.

Ringworm (club lamb fungus, wool rot, and lumpy wool)

Club lamb fungus is a highly contagious fungal infection of the skin of sheep. It is primarily a problem with show lambs that are frequently slick sheared. Club Lamb Fungus is caused by fungus of the genus *Trichophyton*. Infection occurs when the fungus invades the skin and hair (wool) follicles. Fungal spores are transmitted by contaminated clippers, blankets, combs, bedding, bunks, and pens. Lesions can appear anywhere, however, most are found on the head, neck, and back. The infection is susceptible to anti-fungal agents. Club lamb fungus causes a nasty ringworm infection in people.

Ryegrass Staggers

Ryegrass staggers is a disease of grazing animals that causes muscle spasms, loss of muscle control and paralysis. It is caused by a group of toxins that accumulates in the leaf sheaths of perennial ryegrass.

The toxins are produced by a native fungus called ryegrass endophyte, *Neotyphodium lolii*, that grows within the leaves, stems and seeds of perennial ryegrass. Sheep and cattle are most commonly affected but horses, aplaca and deer are also susceptible.

Ryegrass staggers has not been recorded in goats. Affected animals have a stiff gait or are unable to walk. They may injure or kill themselves in transit. The toxins can induce high body temperatures thus animals will try to cool themselves. Younger animals tend to be worst affected. The symptoms of ryegrass staggers usually develop 7-14 days after livestock stock start grazing the toxic parts of the plant. Prolonged exposure to toxic pasture can lead to permanent neurological damage.

Scrapie

Scrapie is a fatal disease affecting the central nervous system of sheep and goats. It is spread from the dam to her offspring and other lambs (and kids) that come into contact with her birthing fluids, placenta, and bedding soiled with birthing fluids. There is not treatment for scrapie. Affected animals always die.

While the occurrence of scrapie in the U.S. sheep flock is low, it is a disease of regulatory concern. This is because scrapie is a member of a family of diseases called "transmissible spongiform encephalopathies (TGE's), which also includes chronic wasting disease (in mule deer and elk), mad cow disease (bovine spongiform encephalopathy) and classic and new variant Creutzfeldt-Jacob's Disease (in humans).

Producers of breeding stock are encouraged to enrolled in the voluntary scrapie flock certification program, which after five years of scrapie-free monitoring, enables a flock to be certified "scrapie-free." Furthermore, while scrapie is not a genetic disease, a sheep's genetic make-up influences its susceptibility to scrapie if exposed to the infective agent. Therefore, sheep can be tested for scrapie resistance.

Scrotal Hernia

A scrotal hernia is when the ram's intestines slip through the inguinal rings into the scrotum. The condition causes an enlargement of the scrotum. Scrotal hernias may be congenital or acquired. They are thought to be caused by trauma. It is not known if genetics plays a role. While it may be possible to surgically repair a scrotal hernia, a more practical option would be harvest them for meat. Obviously, rams with scrotal hernias should not be used for breeding.

Soremouth (contagious ecthyma, scabby mouth, pustular dermatitis, orf)

Soremouth is the most common skin disease affecting sheep (and goats). It is a highly contagious viral infection that can also produce painful human infections. The virus causes scab formation on the skin, usually around the mouth, nostrils, eyes, mammary gland and vulva. It first appears as tiny red nodules, usually at the junction of the lips. Treatment is usually unrewarding. The disease will usually run its course in 1 to 4 weeks.

Effective vaccines are available. The vaccine is applied to a woolless area in the inside of the ear or under a leg where it cannot spread to the mouths of other animals. Once the vaccine is used on the premises, it should be continued yearly. Flocks that have not experienced soremouth should probably not vaccinate for soremouth, since the vaccine introduces the virus to the farm.

Clostridial Diseases

Clostridial diseases are caused by bacteria that occur widely innatureóin soil, sewage, water and in the gut of animals. Theycause a wide range of signs and effects. Whenever animals die afterbeing sick for a short time or are suddenly found dead these diseases should be suspected.

Factors that Can Lead to Disease

- Changes from poor to good food: animals that are placed on lush green pastures after the winter or are suddenly fed rich feeds, such as maize, are at risk
- Lack of care with procedures such as castration, tail docking, wound cleaning and treatment as well as helping animals to lamb or calve can lead to disease
- Stress: any abnormal situation, such as sheep lambing in small camps, is dangerous
- Animals nibbling on carcasses or old bones, or drinking water, or eating feed contaminated by dead animals.

Sudden Death with or Without Gut Signs

- Animals that suffer from these diseases are usually found dead without any visible signs
- Some animals may show signs of stomach pain, depression, watery grey or bloody diarrhoea, weakness and even nervous signs such as convulsion (fits) or paralysis
- Mostly young animals are affected, but older animals may also become sick and die.

Signs in Dead Animals

- Gas-filled red intestines (note that animals that have been dead for a while may show similar signs)
- Soft, pale kidneys (pulpy kidney) Changes in nutrition, stressful times or procedures, deworming Care with change in feed, good management, vaccination

Swollen Legs, Heads and Sudden Death

Common names of diseases in this category are blackquarter (*sponssiekte*), swollen head (*dikkop*) and malignant oedema.

Cattle, Sheep and Goats

- Animals are usually found dead without signs
- The part of the body affected may be very swollen. When the area is touched it feels spongy and is filled with gas bubbles

- Other signs are lameness, depression and swellings as a result of fluid under the skin (oedema)
- Parts of the body are swollen
- Affected muscle has a streaky dark red, greyish-red to yellow and black colour and is filled with gas bubbles
- Wounds from fighting
- The disease develops within 1 to 3 weeks after a wound or a procedure not performed correctly
- The third eyelid moves across the eye
- The animal becomes increasingly stiff and walks with difficulty.
- Death occurs within 1 to 3 days

Signs in Live Animals

- Animals do not have a temperature and may be partially or totally paralysed
- The tongue may hang out of the mouth but the animals will still try to eat. Because they cannot swallow, water given carelessly in the mouth may get into the lungs
- Cattle may die suddenly. Animals die of pneumonia or they stop breathing because of the paralysis
- Sheep may have an arched back, with a drooping head and neck.

Contributing Factors

Contaminated feed and water (dead rats and birds in the feed or water), pica (animals chewing or licking bones or rocks, especially during the dry season and in areas where there is a phosphorus deficiency of the soil), and feeding chicken litter.

Phosphorus supplementation in licks, clean feed and water, vaccination, removing carcasses from the veld.

Diseases with Similar Signs

Clostridial diseases can be confused with one another, as well as with anthrax, toxic plant poisoning, snakebites, poisoning with chemicals, rabies, three-day stiff sickness, redwater, heartwater, infection of the brain, tick paralysis, twin lamb disease (*domsiekte*) and tapeworm cysts in the brain.

Diagnosis

To determine the disease a postmortem should be done, and this may involve laboratory testing to identify the bacteria and toxin. Samples must be collected as soon as possible after death. Ask your animal health technician or state veterinarian to collect the samples and send them to the laboratory.

Treatment

Because these diseases start suddenly with few signs, treatment is nearly always too late to cure the animal. Supportive treatment and antibiotics, such as penicillin, may help in early cases. Treatment of tetanus and botulism is difficult, with poor results. In the early stages, treatment with a substance called antitoxin against the disease may save the animal, but it has to be given as soon as signs are noticed and is not always at hand at times when it may be needed.

Flock Vaccinations

Vaccinations are an important part of a flock health management program. They provide inexpensive "insurance" against diseases that can commonly affect sheep and lambs.

Clostridial Diseases

On most farms, the only universally-recommended vaccine for sheep and lambs is the CD-T toxoid. The CD-T toxid provides three-way protection against enterotoxemia caused by *Clostridium perfringins* types C and D and tetanus (lockjaw) caused by *Clostridium tetani*. There are 7 and 8-way clostridal vaccines that provide protection against additional clostridial diseases, such as blackleg and malignant edema, but the extra protection is often not necessary.

Type C

Enterotoxemia type C, also called hemorrhagic enteritis or "bloody scours," affects lambs mostly during their first few weeks of life, causing a bloody infection in the small intestine. Type C enterotoxemia is often related to indigestion and is predisposed by a change in feed, such as beginning creep feeding or a sudden increase in the milk supply, perhaps caused by the loss of a littermate. The only way to protect lambs from type C enterotoxmia is to vaccinate their dams during late pregnancy.

Type D

Enterotoxemia type D, also called "classic" overeating disease or "pulpy kidney disease," usually affects lambs over one month of age.

Usually it is the largest, fastest growing lamb(s) in the flock that are affected. Type D overeating disease is usually precipitated by a sudden change in feed that causes the bacteria, already present in the lamb's gut, to proliferate, resulting in a toxic, usually fatal reaction. Type D is most commonly observed in lambs that are consuming high concentrate diets, but can also occur in lambs nursing heavy milking dams.

Passive Immunity

To confer passive immunity to lambs through the colostrum (first milk), ewes should be vaccinated with the CD-T toxoid approximately 4 weeks prior to lambing. Ewes lambing for the first time should be vaccinated twice in late pregnancy, four weeks apart. Maternal antibodies will protect lambs for six to eight weeks so long as lambs consume adequate amounts of colostrum. It is recommended that a lamb consume colostrum in the amount of 10 percent of its body weight.

Lambs

Lambs should receive their first CD-T vaccination when they are approximately 6 to 8 weeks of age, followed by a booster 4 weeks later. If pastured animals are later brought into confinement or dry lot for concentrate feeding, a third vaccination should be given. Lambs whose dams were not vaccinated for C and D can be vaccinated with some success at two to three days of age and again in two weeks. However, later vaccinations will likely be more effective, as colostral antibodies usually interfere with vaccinations at very young ages. The lamb's immature immune system may also not be able to respond to vaccination at such a young age. A better alternative may be to vaccinate offspring from non-vaccinated dams when they are approximately 4 weeks of age, followed by a booster 4 weeks later. Anti-toxins can provide immediate short-term immunity if dams were not vaccinated or in the event of disease outbreak or vaccine failure.

Feeder Lambs

Purchased feeder lambs should be vaccinated for type D enterotoxeia at the time of purchase and 2 to 4 weeks later. Feeder lambs purchased as 4-H or FFA projects should receive two type D vaccinations, if they were not vaccinated at the farm of origin.

Tetanus

Lambs whose dams were not vaccinated for tetanus should be given the tetanus anti-toxin at the time of docking and castrating, especially if elastrator bands are used. An antitoxin provides immediate short-term immunity. If a tetanus toxoid product is administered at the time of docking or castrating, it will not provide adequate immunity, as toxoids take 10 days to 2 weeks to provide immunity and require a booster for complete immunity.

Rams and pet sheep should be boostered annually with the CD-T toxoid. As with ewes, they require two vaccinations the first time they are vaccinated.

Other Diseases

In addition to clostridial diseases, there are other diseases for which producers may wish to vaccinate. The use of additional vaccines depends upon the health status of the flock, the perceived disease risk of the flock, and prevalance of diseases in the geographic area where the flock is located. In the U.S. (for sheep), there are approved vaccines for sore mouth, foot rot, caseous lymphadenitis, abortion, *e. coli* scours, parainfluenza-3 (PI-3), epididymitis, and rabies. Vaccines that are not approved for sheep are also sometimes used.

Soremouth

There is an approved vaccine for soremouth (contagious ecthyma, orf), a viral skin disease commonly affecting sheep and goats. The vaccine is live. It causes sore mouth infection (lesions) at a location (on the animal) and time of the producer's choosing. Ewes should be vaccinated well in advance of lambing. Show animals should be vaccinated well in advance of the first show.

To use the vaccine, a woolless area on the animal is scarified, and the rehydrated vaccine is applied to the spot with a brush or similar applicator. Ewes can be vaccinated inside the ear or under the tail. Lambs can be vaccinated inside the thigh. Because the sore mouth vaccine is a live vaccine and sore mouth is highly contagious to humans, care must be taken when applying the vaccine. Gloves should be worn.

Flocks which are free from soremouth should probably not be vaccinated because the soremouth vaccine will introduce the virus to the flock/premises. Once soremouth vaccination is begun, it should be continued annually.

Footrot

Footrot is one of the most ubiquitous and economically devastating diseases in the sheep industry. It causes considerable economic loss due to the costs associated with treating it and the premature culling of carrier animals. There are two vaccines for footrot and foot scald in sheep: Footvax® 10 Strain and Volar™ Footrot Bacterin.

Neither vaccine prevents the diseases from occurring, but when used in conjunction with other management practices such as selection/culling, regular foot trimming, foot soaking/bathing, etc., vaccinations can help reduce infection levels. Footrot vaccines should be administered every 3 to 6 months, prior to anticipated outbreaks of hoof problems (i.e. prior to the wet/rainy season).

Abscesses (at the injection site) are not uncommon with the foot rot vaccines. The limitation of foot rot vaccines is that they might not include the strain of foot rot that is present in a particular flock.

Caseous Lymphadenitis (CL)

There is a vaccine for caseous lymphadenitis in sheep. CL affects primarily the lymphatic system and results in the formation of abscesses in the lymph nodes. It is highly contagious. When it affects the internal organs, it evolves into a chronic wasting disease.

The cost of CL to the sheep industry is probably grossly underestimated. The CLA vaccine is convenient to use because it is combined with CD-T. Vaccination will reduce the number of abscesses in the flock, but it will not prevent the disease from occuring.

Abortion

Abortion is when a female loses her offspring during pregnancy or gives birth to stillborn, weak, or deformed lambs. There are vaccines (individual and combination) for several of the infectious causes of abortion in sheep: enzootic (EAE/*Chlamydia* sp.) and vibriosis (*Campylobacter fetus*).

Abortion vaccines should be administered prior to breeding. Ewes being vaccinated for the first time should receive a second vaccination (booster) in mid-pregnancy. Producers with problem flocks may consider giving a booster as well. Risk factors for abortion include an open flock and/or a history of abortions in the flock. Unfortunately, there is no vaccine (available in the U.S.) for toxoplasmosis, another common cause of abortion in sheep. Since the disease-causing organism is carried by domestic cats, the best protection is to control the farm's cat population by spaying/neutering and keeping cats from contaminating feed sources.

Epididymitis

Epididymitis is a major cause of reduced fertility in rams from western range states. There are vaccines for epididymitis (*Brucella ovis*), but none are deemed fully effective. In addition, vaccination interferes with the ability to eliminate infected rams from the flock, as vaccinated rams will test positive for *B. ovis*.

E.Coli *Scours*

Scours in baby lambs can be caused by *E. coli*. There is a vaccine that can be administered to ewes at the same time as CD-T to pass immunity to lambs through the colostrum. An alternative to vaccination is to give newborn lambs oral *E. coli* antibody at birth.

Rabies

Though the risk to sheep is usually minimal, rabies vaccination may be advised if the flock is located in a rabies-infected area, the animals are valuable, and livestock have access to wooded areas or areas frequented by raccoons, skunks, foxes, or other known carriers of rabies. Frequent interaction with livestock may be another reason to consider vaccinating.

The cost of the rabies vaccine relative to the value of the animals should be considered. The large animal rabies vaccine is approved for use in sheep. Producers should consult their veterinarian regarding rabies vaccination. Some states require rabies vaccination for exhibition at fairs and shows. All dogs and cats on the farm should be vaccinated against rabies.

Autogenous Vaccines

When no commercial vaccine is available, autogenous or custom vaccines can be made. They are usually made from bacteria or viruses that have been isolated on a farm in conjunction with a disease. Autogenous vaccines are usually not as effective as commercial vaccines.

Giving Vaccines

Most vaccines are given subcutaneously (sub-Q), i.e. under the skin. Some vaccines are given intramuscularly (IM). Occasionally, some are given topically (e.g. sore mouth) or intranasally (e.g. Nasalgen®). For subcutaneous vaccines, use a 1/2 or 3/4 inch, 18- or 20-gauge needle. Subcutaneous vaccinations can be given over the ribs, behind the armpit, or high up on the neck. The needle used to withdraw vaccine from the bottle should not be the same needle used to inject the animal.

In order for vaccination programs to be successful, label directions should be carefully followed. Vaccines should be stored, handled, and administered properly. Only healthy sheep and lambs should be vaccinated. It is also important to note that vaccines have limitations and that the immunity imparted by vaccines can sometimes by inadequate or overwhelmed by disease challenge.

Future Vaccines

With the increasing role of small ruminants in small farms and sustainable farming systems, hopefully animal health companies will develop and license more vaccines for sheep.

Scientists are currently working to develop vaccines to protect small ruminants against *Haemonchus contortus* and other gastro-intestinal and blood-sucking parasites. The research is promising. Thus far, the challenge has been developing effective vaccines using recombinant DNA technology, as other methods of vaccine generation are not economically feasible.

Not Vaccinating

Many sheep producers will tell you that they never vaccinate. Other producers vaccinate for diseases which are not a high risk. Vaccination is a form of risk management. Each producer must weights the pros and cons of vaccinating for a specific disease. If the cost of vaccination excees the expected losses, then vaccination is probably not cost-effective. Conversely, if expected losses exceed the cost of vaccination, they vaccination is a good risk management tool.

At the same time, it is not advisable to wait until you have a disease outbreak before instituting a vaccination program. The risk of a disease outbreak should be the criteria that is used to determine the need for vaccination. A producer's tolerence for risk will also come into play.

Livestock Diseases and the Traditional Medicine

Ethnobotanical inquiries were carried out from 1980 to 1990 to collect plants used in both veterinary and human medicines. A description of livestock diseases is made and the plant material formulas used for their treatment are inventoried. Vernacular and scientific names, parts of the plant used and instructions for use are reported. About 31 groups representing 62 vernacular names of animal diseases have been recorded and translated into English and French languages, and 124 plant species for treatment of livestock diseases identified. Plant materials are usually prescribed as maceration, infusion or decoction to be taken orally or by rectal administration and by application of ashes loco denti in the scarifications made on the ailing part of the body. Plant material is used singly or in combination. People say that the combination of several ingredients increase the chance of recovery. Moreover, a disease can be cured by one or more medicinal formulas and one formula can be used for the treatment of several diseases.

Introduction

Through several inquiries in the Bushi area about the inventory of medicinal plants (Chifundera, 1993), it has been observed that native healers practise both veterinary and human medicines. Thus it has been possible to record medicaments used for the treatment of livestock diseases.

Study Area

The Bushi area has been described in previous papers (Chifundera, 1992). Briefly, the Bushi is a wide territory of 8,192 km2 located on the Western and Southern shores of Lake Kivu (28°30'-29°E and 1°30'-3°S). The Bashi tribe is of Bantu origin and its population is presently estimated to about 1,200,000 inhabitants (124 inhab/km2). Mashi is vernacular language which belongs to the D. 50 zone of Guthrie's linguistic classification (Guthrie, 1967). The equatorial climate of the study area is temperate owing to its high altitude which varies between 900 and 3,308 m. Subalpine meadow covers all the region and an abundand vegetation grows on the rich volcanic and ferraltic soils.

Agriculture is the predominant livelihood but pasture land have decreased because of demographic increase. The number of cattle per household varies from 5 to 10 heads (Paluku, 1984). Many factors explain the animal productivity such as shortage of land, forage and budget, lack of farming education and mainly the livestock diseases which annually cause a mortality rate to vary between 19.6 and 35% (Paluku, 1984; Kambaza, et al., 1985; Ntumba, 1990). In regard to the higher rate of mortality, the intervention of veterinary medicine appears to be of great importance.

Material and Methods

Ethnobotanical inquiries were carried out from 1980 to 1990 to collect plants for in both veterinary and human medicines. Traditional healers, cattle-breeders, shepherds and households were interviewed: each of them were asked to mention all known diseases with their symptoms and when possible, show real examples. Blood and stool samples of sick animals were collected for laboratory analysis at Lwiro (Democratic Republic of Congo) in the Laboratory of Veterinary

Medicine. A modern veterinarian visited the suffering animals to make a diagnosis through direct observations. Results from the laboratory were also used to identify the diseases. Vernacular names of livestock diseases and medicinal plants were recorded as well as the instruction for use of drugs.

Each disease or group of diseases was described by giving the vernacular, English and French names and the symptoms observed by the healers or by the households. It has been observed that a symptom can represent more than one disease. People group the diseases by the same symptoms, and consequently, apply the same treatment method to the disease of a group.

When people cannot exactly recognise any difference of symptoms, a modern veteririan has helped to differentiate the diseases and a vernacular name was given. The vernacular name used in the identification of an unknown microbial disease can be ambiguous. In such cases, a modern veterinarian is of great importance in identifying the illness: classic bacteriological methods (Dumas, *et al.*, 1951) were used and microscopic examinations of stools and haematological tests were made to determine the diseases in question.

For the collected samples of medicinal plants, vernacular names and the plant part used were recorded. All the vernacular names were of the Mashi language (Guthrie, 1967). However, plant samples were scientifically identified by reference to the Herbarium of the Laboratory of Botany, Department of Biology at Lwiro (Democratic Republic of Congo) where voucher specimens are preserved.

Results

About 31 groups representing 62 vernacular names of animal diseases have been recorded and translated into English and French languages (Appendices 1, 2, 3).

Chifundera

People refer to external apparent symptoms to nominate a disease which can have several causes. The diseases with the same symptoms are grouped together despite their different causes or effects and people use the same medicinal formula for their treatment. A compilation of 124 plant species used for the treatment of livestock diseases (Appendix 4) have been made. People use the same treatment method for all animal species (cow, goat, sheep, hen). When an animal is ill, the household looks for medicaments by consulting a native healer. Plant materials are usually prescribed as maceration, infusion or decoction to be administered orally or rectally and by application of ashes loco denti in the scarifications made on the ailing part of the body. Plant material is used singly or in combination. People say that the combination of several ingredients increase the chance of recovery. Moreover, a disease can be cured by one or more medicinal formulas and one formula can be used for the treatment of several diseases.

Discussion and Conclusion

This study records the indigenous knowledge on the farming activities in the Bushi area. The results obtained from intensive inquiries reveal interesting aspects of the traditional methods for the treatment of livestock diseases, provide a basis of a design concept toward structuring and improving the problems which the Bushi farming activities face (Schmitz, 1985). Cattle is used in economic transactions and social exchanges to cover the dowry and to maintain relationship between members of the social groups in heritage, payment of tenure and to preserve the honour for belonging to the higher social rank. But the income from husbandry is expected if the animals are in a good health conditions. For this reason, people have developed a range of methods for the treatment of livestock diseases.

The efficacy of all medicinal formulas mentioned in the treatment methods is not yet ascertained. But the collection of pharmacognosical data from this study can provide a basis for the integration of folk uses in the conventional veterinary medicine. This is to say that traditional medicine can be a real source for insights into material from which the discovery of new compounds of medicinal values may be made (Farnsworth et al., 1986; Akerele, 1984, 1988, 1992; Gujar, 1990; Galeffi & Marini-Bettolo, 1988). For this, phytochemical screening and biological assays of plant drugs must be carried out to display the active principles (Gujar, 1990). The laboratory work is in progress to evaluate the efficacy of some plant extracts: antibacterial, antivenomous, anthelminthic, acaricidal, antiparasitic and molluscicidal plants are under evaluation in laboratory conditions (Chifundera, et al., 1993). Some substances, such as alkaloids, tannins, lignans, saponins, quinons, phenols, phytoecdysons and various glycosides have been isolated and pointed out as substances which are endowed with biological activities (Chifundera, et al., 1993; Scalbert, 1991).

Notifiable Diseases

There are a number of diseases in animals that are notifiable. If a producer suspects or can confirm that an animal is showing symptoms of a notifiable disease it must be reported to a local vet or by contacting the Emergency Animal Disease Watch Hotline on 1800 675 888.

Principles of Herd or Flock Health

Producers should take a proactive approach to managing the health of their herd or flock by:

- Learning about the common cattle, sheep or goat diseases that occur locally.
- Aiming for prevention rather than treatment.
- Identifying historic sites or sites of old yards and stock routes on the property that may be potential sources of disease.
- Developing a herd or flock disease management plan to manage the health of animals already on the farm and to prevent introduced stock bringing new diseases onto the farm.
- Using an appropriate combination of management, preventative treatments, vaccination and curative treatments to manage the health of the herd or flock.
- Improving nutrition to allow livestock to develop an effective immune response to diseases.
- Vaccinating against diseases for which vaccines are available and cost-effective.
- Quarantining all introduced livestock to prevent the introduction of new diseases.
- Monitoring the health and welfare of livestock as frequently as practical.
- Promptly treating or euthanising any animals suffering from disease.
- Quarantining carcases of any animals that die suddenly, unexpectedly or for unknown reasons.
- Seeking veterinary advice for any unexplained health problems.

Use of Veterinary Products

When it is necessary to use veterinary products, such as antibiotics, vaccines or other chemicals to prevent or treat diseases in livestock, producers should:

- Read the label thoroughly before use.

- Observe all label restrictions and follow all label directions for dose rates, safety precautions, personal protective equipment, withholding periods (WHPs), export slaughter intervals (ESIs), re-handling intervals and disposal of empty containers and unused product.
- Follow any specific instructions provided by their veterinarian.
- Record the appropriate information and include on the if the stock are sold.

Infectious

Infectious diseases can be caused by bacteria, fungi or viruses.

Infectious diseases of cattle, sheep and goats in Australia that can lead to significant economic loss include:

- Bovine respiratory disease
- Calf scours
- Cheesy gland
- Clostridial diseases
- Footrot
- Johne's disease
- Leptospirosis
- Pestivirus
- Pinkeye
- Three day sickness
- Vibriosis
- Trichomoniasis.

Notifiable Diseases

Some infectious diseases are also 'notifiable diseases'. If a producer suspects or can confirm that an animal is showing symptoms of a notifiable disease it must be reported to a local vet or the Emergency Animal Disease Watch Hotline on 1800 675 888.

The Department of Agriculture, Fisheries and Forestry maintains a national list and state and territory lists of notifiable animal diseases.

Risks and Risk Management

Some infectious diseases have highly visible consequences, while others remain silent for weeks or months. Where, in the absence of a drought or seasonal feed shortage, there has been a dramatic change in the condition of animals, producers should suspect that disease is present and arrange for veterinary investigations to be carried out.

With all diseases and nutritional deficiencies, assess the risk based on previous local district history by seeking local information from veterinarians, state government officers and consultants, and if available, the property history.

Many infectious diseases of cattle, sheep and goats do not occur in Australia and it is important to keep these diseases out of Australia, farm and industry biosecurity plans help ensure this. Information on biosecurity plans for diseases such as Foot and Mouth Disease, Bovine Spongiform Encephalopathy and Scrapie can be found on the

Poisonings

The main potential sources of poisonings for livestock on farm are:

- Chemicals
  - o Veterinary chemicals and drugs used to treat animals.
  - o Chemical residues on fodder crops or pastures.
  - o Old dip sites and yards.
  - o Waste (machinery, batteries, used chemical containers) left lying around on farms.
- Overdoses
  - o Through veterinary chemicals and drugs.
- Toxic plants
  - o A variety of plants can have toxic effects on livestock.

Common Cattle Diseases and Treatments

There are many common cattle diseases that occur in eastern North Carolina cow/calf herds. Below is a discussion of two of these diseases, possible treatments, and advice on veterinary care.

Pinkeye

Pinkeye is one of the most common diseases in cattle. It can affect all ages of cattle and it is highly contagious. Multiple strains of bacteria can cause the disease, and it can be difficult to determine which one is the culprit in your herd. In the early stages of pinkeye, the animal will be very sensitive to light, and you may see a bluish spot on the lens of the eye, followed by watery discharge. Once the animal has pinkeye, it will be bothered easily by vectors such as flies, dust, and tall grass seedheads.

Treating Pinkeye

Pinkeye can be treated with over the counter medication such as LA-200 or penicillin. If these treatments do not improve the eye, a vet should tend to the eye in order for the animal to recover. Over the counter treatments or home remedies that involve powder, sprays, or salt should not be used due to the irritating nature of these products.

Cancer eye should not be confused with pinkeye, since cancer eye is much more serious and usually is first noticed by lumps or bumps growing around the eye. Animals with cancer eye or pinkeye should not be taken to a stockyard in order to safeguard the human food supply and prevent other animals from contracting the diseases.

Calf Diarrhea/Scours

Calf scours is one of the most common diseases in newborn calves. Contrary to popular belief, it is impossible to tell what bacteria is affecting the animal based solely on the colour of the feces. However, a good guess can be made about the possible bacteria present based on other factors. If the scours occurs in a calf less than 10 days old, the bacteria present is probably E. Coli, Rotavirus, or Coronavirus. Cryptosporidium is a protozoa that can cause scours in calves at 5-35 days of age.

Salmonella is severe bloody diarrhea and a high body temperature. Calves less than 21 days old will not be troubled by Coccidia because of the incubation period of the disease in the calf's body. When treating calf scours, it is important for the animal to continue to drink (or be forced to drink) milk to prevent further dehydration and provide adequate nutrition. Because of the diarrhea, metabolic acidosis may occur which will cause the animal to breathe heavily. If the calf is lying on the ground and willing to accept your intervention, then it should be treated. If the animal readily gets up to follow its mother, even with diarrhea, then it will most likely recover quickly.

Treating Calf Scours (Clell V. Bagley, DVM, Extension Veterinarian, Utah State University):

> *There are a variety of fluid and electrolyte formulas available and most will work to some extent. Consult with your veterinarian about his choice and why. If the products are not working, re-evaluate with him again. Some formulas also contain a gel substance which helps to add bulk and may absorb some toxins (poisons) from the gut. Most calves with scours tend to be acidotic (their*

system is too acid). It will help these calves to receive
electrolytes that are alkaline (basic) in nature for 24–36
hours. After that they should be changed to non-alkaline
electrolytes.

If being used with or near milk feeding, an acetate form should
be used. If this is not a problem them bicarbonate or lactate can be
used. The use of systemic antibiotics by injection may also be of benefit
if a bacterial infection has become generalised in the calf's body. The
major problem encountered in treatment with fluids and electrolytes
is that producers give too little, too late. Plan to give 2 qts., 2–4 times
per day.

Determine the frequency of treatment needed by the amount of
dehydration present; this is evidenced by sinking of the eyes and
elasticity of skin on the neck and withers. Don't mix the fluid and
electrolytes with milk; that prevents curd formation and the milk is
then of no benefit. If you are feeding milk, wait for 15–20 minutes
before giving the fluid and elect

Vaccination of Farm Animals

What Diseases can Vaccination Prevent?

Vaccination protects hundreds of millions of animals worldwide
from disease and possibly death.

Animals, just like humans, suffer from a range of infectious
diseases. As veterinary medicine has advanced, prevention of disease
has become a priority as healthy food comes from healthy animals.
One of the best means of preventing disease is by creating immunity
in the animal. This is usually achieved by vaccination.

The principle of vaccination has been established for over 200
years. Since those early days, enormous strides have been made in
the development of vaccines, which have helped to prevent and in
some cases eliminate many diseases in humans, farm animals and the
family pet.

Animals which develop disease often require treatment with
medicines so vaccination helps reduce the amount of pharmaceuticals
used in the treatment of animals. Vaccination presents no hazard to
consumers of produce from vaccinated animals.

Not all animals need every vaccine. Some, like clostridial disease
prevention, are basically routine, just like childhood vaccination
programmes. The vaccination programme chosen for farm animals
depends on the management system, the location of the farm and the

history of the herd or flock (and whether or not a disease is likely to be encountered). Most farm animals are young, and these animals (just like children) are often more susceptible to infection. So, for example, calves often need to be protected by vaccination against respiratory disease. Some of the diseases that can be prevented are shown below.

Species Diseases Controlled by Vaccines in the Uk

Cattle Blackleg, tetanus, 'husk' (lungworm disease), rotavirus, infectious bovine rhinotracheictis (IBR), respiratory syncytial virus, pasteurellosis, enteritis, leptospirosis, mastitis, ringworm, BVD, PI3, coronavirus, salmonella, E Coli. Sheep (& goats)Clostridial diseases (8 different species including tetanus), pasteurellosis, ovine abortion (chlamydiosis and toxoplasmosis), louping ill, contagious pustular dermatitis (orf), footrot. Pigs Erysipelas, parvovirus, colibacillosis, clostridial disease, atrophic rhinitis, enteritis, porcine pneumonia, PRRS.

Poultry Avian coccidiosis, avian encephalomyelitis, avian infectious bronchitis, avian infectious bursal disease, avian reovirus, chicken anaemia virus, duck virus enteritis, egg drop syndrome 1976, erysipelas, infectious laryngotracheitis, Marek's disease, Newcastle disease, pasteurellosis, post-natal colibacillosis, salmonellosis, swollen head syndrome, turkey haemorrhagic enteritis, turkey rhinotracheitis

Fish Enteric redmouth disease, furunculosis, vibriosis (vibrio anguillarum, vibrio salmonicida and Vibrio viscosus (now named moratella viscosus))

How Do Vaccines Work?

Vaccines stimulate the body to produce its own defence against infection. Mimicking what happens when an animal has been exposed to disease, the body and its defensive system will "remember" the identity of the invading organisms. So, when the animal comes into contact with a disease, its body is ready to fight it and the animal will not fall ill and suffer. This protects the individual animal and because this animal will not develop the disease and will not become infective, it will also help protect the population from the disease - "herd immunity".

A vaccine may consist of live but attenuated viruses or bacteria, or killed (inactivated) viruses or bacteria, or parts of them.

"Killed" or inactivated vaccines are prepared from killed organisms or fractions of the organism incapable of causing disease. They generally provide a relatively short period of immunity.

In attenuated vaccines, the immunising agent (antigen) is an organism such as a virus, bacterium or parasite, which has been developed to stimulate the production of the appropriate antibodies without causing the disease. Live vaccines are particularly effective in providing long-term protection, because they are a more powerful stimulus to the immune system. They are also more versatile in their route of administration.

Biotechnology can provide vaccines for diseases which cannot be controlled by conventional vaccine technology and create more specific, better defined products with even greater safety and efficacy.

Vaccination can be by a wide variety of routes: through water, baits, airspray, eye inoculation, intranasally, orally or using the more classical injection.

Achieving initial immunity may require more than one injection. Once established, this can be boosted by subsequent vaccination, as required. Modern vaccine research and technology means that some vaccines can actively protect against a variety of diseases, in a single product. These are called multivalent vaccines and using these reduces the number of injections, broadens disease protection - and helps reduce costs to the farmer.

How are Vaccines Controlled?

In the early days vaccination was risky. Vaccines were crude, using cultures or suspensions of diseased material treated to reduce infectivity. Some of the impurities in the injection also produced unwanted side effects.

But now, through much development work by vaccine manufacturers, risk from the immunising agent has been decreased while its efficiency has been increased. Present day vaccines are safe and effective, having been designed specifically to avoid side effects and any remaining ability to cause disease. The advent of biotechnology has opened new doors to even more exciting developments.

Whether for disease prevention or treatment, the veterinarian, the animal owner and the public all have a right to expect that the research, development and bringing to market of animal medicines is reliably based on the triple standards of quality, safety and efficacy. The extremely stringent requirements for product registration set down in European law reflect this. If these requirements are not met, a vaccine will not be allowed on the market. Careful monitoring and review of products and disease patterns ensure that once on the market, vaccines remain safe and effective. There are very strict quality control processes to guarantee the safety and efficacy of each dose of vaccine. Today's vaccines are very effective and have a remarkably high safety record. Millions of doses are used annually in the UK alone. The use of vaccines has brought significant levels of control against diseases that farm animals previously suffered.

There is a constant quest for new preventive measures to meet the changing challenges to animal health. Indeed the diseases threatening animals evolve themselves; just like with human influenza, when the medical profession needs to be prepared with a vaccine to counter the particular strain that is prevalent at the time.

So the work goes on, as animal medicine companies continue to look for new vaccines to help farmers protect their animals. Vaccines, when available, provide a safe and effective answer to many animal welfare problems and represent an important field of ongoing research.

Case Studies

Case Study 1: Clostridial Disease in Sheep and Lambs

Clostridia are soil dwelling bacteria that can enter sheep even as they graze. They pose a constant and serious threat to flock health: before the introduction of vaccines they were causing losses of up to 50% of lambs. The potential for this remains. Onset is sudden, death is rapid and there is often no opportunity for successful treatment - flock vaccination provides the only method of control.

Clostridial vaccine manufacturers report that farmers who make mistakes in their vaccination regime - or are prevented by organic production contracts from using the vaccines routinely - can find that sudden and large-scale losses with clostridial diseases such as pulpy kidney or braxy occur.

Luckily clostridial vaccines make this scenario much less common.

Case Study 2: Aujeszky's Disease (pseudorabies)

A serious, frequently fatal, viral infection in pigs, Aujeszky's was a disease that European vets and farmers were determined to eradicate. Pigs that do recover can still carry infection, acting as a risk to others. Because they have had the disease, they bear residual antibodies. Early vaccines contributed to a reduction in disease. However they left vaccinated pigs with antibodies indistinguishable from those in an animal which had recovered from the disease but remained a carrier. So it was impossible to distinguish a vaccinated animal from an infected one.

One option to eradicate the disease involved removing all pigs with antibodies - this was actually used in Great Britain. But the vaccine was redesigned to remove from the vaccine virus the 'gene message' for a non-essential glycoprotein, which is found in all known infective strains of the virus. In parallel, a serological test was developed to accompany this. Now vaccinated animals could be differentiated from those naturally infected. This meant that there was no longer a need to slaughter all pigs with antibodies, and vaccination could play a role in the eradication schemes.

Case Study 3: Newcastle Disease

Newcastle disease is caused by a highly contagious virus that not only affects poultry (chickens in particular) but also can exist in carrier state in wild birds. Although endemic in many countries of the world, the UK has been free of the disease for some years. There is no treatment, but the UK's disease free status is maintained by routine vaccination, usually via the drinking water or by coarse spray, although sometimes intranasal or intraocular vaccines are given.

Case Study 4: Leptospirosis

Leptospirosis occurs in 60% of UK dairy herds, is an important bacterial disease of cattle and can lead to significant economic losses through symptoms as varied as abortion, reproductive failure and loss of milk production. Leptospirosis can also be transmitted from cows to humans where it can cause a flu-like syndrome. Vaccination against leptospirosis will protect cattle from developing the disease and thus economic benefits for the farmer. Vaccination also has human health benefits as it will prevent transmission to farm workers.

Case Study 5: Bovine Respiratory Disease

Calf pneumonia remains one of the most important causes of economic loss to cattle farmers as well as being a cause of suffering to the affected animals. The total cost to farmers in the UK has been estimated to be over £80 million.

Calves suffering from pneumonia can stop eating, lose weight, suffer pain, and in some cases may die. They also require extra nursing and treatment with antibiotics and some cases anti-inflammatory medicines. Even after they recover affected calves are often slow to put on weight and grow properly.

There are a number of triggers of calf pneumonia including management and other facts but the actual causes are a variety of bacteria, viruses and mycoplasmas. Vaccines are now available which will provide effective control of the most common bacterial and viral causes of calf pneumonia. These vaccines are given before high-risk times such as housing and the winter months. This means that there is an improvement in animal welfare as pneumonia is an important cause of suffering in animals, as well as obvious economic benefits for the farmer since the total cost of pneumonia can reach in the order of £80 per affected calf.

Case study 6: Trout Vaccination

Enteric Red Mouth caused by Yersinia ruckeri first entered British trout farming in 1982/3. From the first point of entry it spread rapidly around the country and became an endemic problem causing up to 20 percent mortality even with regular treatments. Immersion vaccination was introduced in 1983 and the severity of the disease was contained but problems persisted particularly as the intensity of production increased. In recent years an oral booster vaccine has been introduced which has enabled trout farmers to produce their fish without significant antibiotic intervention.

Case Study 7: Salmon Vaccination

Furunculosis has been present in wild salmon since the 1800's. With the advent of salmon farming the disease became a serious problem causing significant losses. In the late 1980's the viability of the industry was threatened by this endemic disease problem. The industry invested very heavily with government backing and developed a unique vaccine based upon special antigens linked to the infection mechanisms of the bacteria causing the disease. This vaccine was introduced in the early 1990's and in conjunction with good husbandry measures resulted in a dramatic turn around. Mortalities to the disease are now almost unknown and welfare of the farmed salmon is greatly enhanced.

Controls on Animal Medicines

How does an Animal Medicine Get to the Market?

Before an animal medicine can be sold in the UK it must be approved. This takes the form of a marketing authorisation. The UK has one of the most stringent licensing systems for the authorisation of animal medicines in Europe, if not the world.

Development of a new animal medicine is very lengthy and expensive process. To develop a new product from scratch takes many years and costs millions of pounds.

Once a potentially useful compound has been identified, amongst other things:

- studies have to be done into its pharmacology and modes of action
- studies are carried out into its potential toxicity (both acute and long term: to the animal, the person who will administer the medicine, the consumer of any produce from a treated animal and the environment)
- analytical methods have to be developed to look for any residues left
- dose finding studies are carried out to find out at what dose the substance is effective in the appropriate species
- for farm animal medicines there has to be a Maximum Residue Limit for the active ingredient and residue depletion studies are needed to set withdrawal periods
- production methods have to be devised and scaled up to a commercial production line
- work is done on the formulation of the product
- stability tests are carried out
- field trials are run to test the product in real life.

To apply for the marketing authorisation needed to sell an animal medicine, the company has to put together a very extensive dossier of information, which must follow a predetermined format to set out in European law. This information helps the national or European regulators to carry out an independent scientific assessment of a product's safety, quality and efficacy.

So Who Does the Approving?

There are four routes for obtaining marketing authorisations:

- the National procedure under which applications with supporting data are submitted to the Veterinary Medicines Directorate (VMD), a part of the Department for Environment, Food & Rural Affairs. Marketing authorisations granted under this procedure are valid in the UK only. Only products that are not already authorised anywhere in the EU are eligible for the national procedure.
- the Decentralised and Mutual Recognition procedures are very similar: a holder of a marketing authorisation issued by one

member state may apply to one or more other member states to issue identical authorisations on the basis of "mutual recognition". If a product is not yet authorised anywhere in the EU, an application may be made simultaneously to several member states under the Decentralised Procedure, with one of the member states (the "rapporteur") taking the lead on assessment of the dossier.

If one of the member states concerned considers that the product as authorised constitutes a risk to animal or public health or to the environment, the dossier is referred to the EU Committee for Veterinary Medicinal Products (CVMP) for "arbitration", where a binding decision is reached.

- the Centralised procedure is obligatory for some high technology products and optional for some other products. An application is made to the European Medicines Agency (EMEA). The authorisation, if subsequently granted, is issued by the European Commission and is valid in all member states.

How Do We Know an Animal Medicine is Safe?

A marketing authorisation will only be granted if the veterinarians, pharmacists, chemists, toxicologists and environmental experts, either at the VMD in the UK or EMEA for products seeking EU-wide approach, and their advisory committees of independent experts (the Veterinary Products Committee in the UK or CVMP in Europe), are fully satisfied.

To get the authorisation, it is necessary to prove that the product is safe, that it will work, and that it is of good and consistent quality.

Safety

The safety aspects make sure the medicine can be used safely without causing harm to the animal being treated, people giving the treatment, the environment and, in the case of farm animals, that it will be safe to eat the meat, milk, eggs or honey from animals treated.

For food-producing animals, studies are required to see how quickly residues of the medicine are eliminated from the animal. Maximum Residue Limits (MRLs) are established to set a maximum level of the substance(s) concerned that may remain in the animal without posing a risk to consumers of produce taken from it. Withdrawal periods (the time between administration of the medicine and slaughter or the taking of food produce, eg milk or eggs) are then set to ensure that any remaining residues are below the MRL. Huge safety margins are built into the system to ensure that consumers are not put at risk.

Quality

Quality is very important to ensure that product safety is upheld. The quality assessment makes sure that all batches of a product meet the required standards. Studies of the product's stability are used to ensure that the product retains its full potency, efficacy and safety, even when it is stored for long periods.

Efficacy

All medicines must do what they claim to do when used as instructed on the label. Extensive tests are carried out in the laboratory, in disease challenge studies and in field trials, to make sure that the product will actually work in practical "real life" situations, against the specified disease in the named species of animal, at the dose rate, frequency and duration of treatment recommended, and by the route of administration specified.

Only when the regulator is satisfied on all three criteria does it issue a marketing authorisation, without which the company is not permitted to sell the product.

What Happens Once a Product is on the Market?

Checks do not end at product approval. Although the requirements to prove safety, quality and efficacy are very strict, there is a rigorous system to report any problems experienced with products once they are on the market. Companies are required by law to report to the VMD any side effects they are told about. Vets and other animal medicine users are also actively encouraged to report problems they encounter. This allows any potential problems to be quickly recognised and dealt with.

How is the Distribution of Animal Medicines Controlled?

Distribution of animal medicines in the UK is strictly controlled by a variety of legislation. Wholesalers are required to hold an authorisation appropriate to the type of products in which they are dealing. Manufacturers are required to hold a manufacturer's authorisation for the products they produce, and their premises are regularly inspected – for pharmaceuticals by the Medicines and Healthcare Products Regulatory Agency (an executive agency of the Department of Health) or for vaccines by the Veterinary Medicines Directorate. The inspectors check the premises are suitable for the production of safe, effective medicines of a consistently high quality, and that they are being manufactured in accordance with their marketing authorisations. Vets' and merchants' premises and pharmacies are all regularly inspected to ensure they meet the required standards. All authorised animal medicines are allocated to a specific distribution category, which controls the route through which they can be sold. How do we know there are no harmful residues of animal medicines in our food?

Use of animal medicines in farm animals is strictly controlled by European law and requires observance of the withdrawal period. This is the time which passes between the last dose given to the animal and the time when the level of residues in the tissues (muscle, liver, kidney, skin/fat) or products (milk, eggs, honey) falls below the MRL.

The withdrawal period is set out in the data sheet for the medicine and in the instructions for use which are part of the product packaging. Farmers are required by law to record all uses of animal medicines; it is therefore straightforward to ensure withdrawal periods are observed.

Statistics back this up: in the UK farmers and vets have an excellent track record of observing the regulations – and measures are in place to ensure things to stay that way. As part of that effort, the VMD operates two complementary surveillance programmes for animal medicine residues to ensure that residues above the MRL do not occur and that prohibited or illegal drugs are not used. In the few cases where confirmatory analysis shows presence of unauthorised medicines or concentrations above the MRL, these are followed up. The State Veterinary Service investigates the farm, advises, inspects and if appropriate, prosecutes.

The Veterinary Residues Committee independently scrutinises the surveillance for veterinary residues in the UK. They publish their summary results in their Annual Report. Results are reassuring. Of almost 40,000 analyses annually, only a handful (less than 0.2%) contain detectable residues of authorised veterinary medicinal products at concentrations above the relevant MRL, and the independent Committee concludes that these pose no risk to consumers.

Maximum Residue Limits (MRLs) and the Safety of Food from Animals

Residues of veterinary medicinal products, as defined by the European Union, are "pharmacologically active substances (whether active principles, excipients or degradation products) and their metabolites which remain in foodstuffs obtained from animals to which the veterinary medicinal product in question has been administered".

An MRL is the maximum concentration of residue following administration of a veterinary medicine which is legally permitted or acceptable in food under the laws of the EU.

The responsibility for keeping residues under the MRL lies with veterinary surgeons and farmers, using licensed animal medicines.

Use of animal medicines is strictly controlled by European law, and requires observance of the withdrawal period. This is the time which passes between the last dose given to the animal and the time when the level of residues in the tissues (muscle, liver, kidney, skin/fat) or products (milk, eggs, honey) is lower than or equal to the MRL. Until the withdrawal period has elapsed, the animal or its products must not be used for human consumption.

The withdrawal period is set out in the data sheet for the medicine and in the instructions for use which are part of the product packaging. Farmers are required by law to record all uses of animal medicines; it is therefore straightforward to ensure that withdrawal periods are observed.

Withdrawal periods exist so that MRLs are not exceeded and to ensure consumer safety. Accordingly, safety is of paramount importance when both MRLs and withdrawal periods are established and the legislators always err on the side of caution. As a result, although residues above the MRL should not occur, even if they do, they generally present no risk to the consumer because of the very large safety margins used in setting the MRL.

For example, the calculation of the MRL value is based on the acceptable daily intake (ADI) for the drug in question. The calculation of the ADI includes an extremely large safety factor. In addition, the MRL calculation assumes an average intake per person of 500g of meat (over a pound!), 1.5 litres of milk (over 2.5 pints!), 2 eggs and 20g (nearly an ounce) of honey. Legislators might be well advised to consider the health implications for obesity and cholesterol levels!

Residues Surveillance

In the UK, farmers and veterinarians have an excellent track record of observing the regulations - and measures are in place to ensure things stay that way. As part of that effort, the Veterinary

Medicines Directorate (VMD) operates two complementary surveillance programmes for residues of veterinary drugs in food of animal origin to ensure that residues above the MRL do not occur and that prohibited or illegal drugs are not being used:

Statutory Programme

A statutory programme fulfils the UK's obligations under Directive 96/23/EC. This Directive extended the previous statutory residues testing programme to poultry and aquaculture (salmon and trout), eggs, wild and farmed game and honey, and changed the previous regime for red meat by requiring a higher number of samples to be taken on farm with a consequent reduction in sampling at slaughterhouses.

Each year samples are collected from randomly selected farms and abattoirs by the State Veterinary Service (SVS) and the Meat Hygiene Service and analyses performed. In 2003 there were some 30 975 samples collected and 35 399 analyses performed. Analysis is carried out by the Laboratory of the Government Chemist and results are published by the Veterinary Medicines Directorate quarterly, and annually by the Veterinary Residues Committee (VRC). The results are presented for independent scrutiny at meetings of the VRC during the year. All the results are also seen by the Food Standards Agency. They can give a scientific opinion on the significance for human health.

In 2003 the VRC said that overall, the results of the National Surveillance Scheme indicate that the UK authorised uses of veterinary medicinal products did not result in residues of human health concern.

Follow-up action is taken by the State Veterinary Service on every sample which on confirmatory analysis shows the presence of unauthorised substances or concentrations of authorised substances above the MRL. A thorough on-farm investigation is carried out, with farmers advised how to avoid residues of veterinary medicines entering the food chain. If inspection of farm records and stock and the taking of further samples reveals clear evidence of abuse, the farmer will be prosecuted.

Non-Statutory Programme

A non-statutory programme supplements and complements the National Surveillance Scheme, extending residue analysis to imported and processed foods. It gives valuable information on foods that do not fall within the NSS.

Samples are taken from popular presentations of meat and animal products, collected from shops and at the border inspection posts. Samples are subjected to a range of analyses by the Central Science Laboratory in York. In 2003, there were 5468 analyses, targeted in particular foods where intelligence had suggested the possible presence of banned substances being used as veterinary medicines.

Retailers are informed by VMD of any "positive" samples purchased from their stores, and consumer organisations, local authorities, relevant trade associations and producers are contacted where appropriate to make them aware of the results.

If the products are imported, the SVS will contact the Chief Veterinary Officer of the country concerned. There are powers under the Food Safety Act to remove from the food chain food products containing residues at concentrations which represent a danger to human health.

In addition to these schemes, milk is tested for antibiotic residues by the dairy companies and heavy penalties face dairy farmers whose milk fails to meet the necessary requirements. Food retailers and processors also frequently carry out their own checks.

How MRLs are Set ?

Maximum Residue Limits are set by the European Commission after adoption by the Standing Committee, following an opinion of the Committee for Veterinary Medicinal Products (CVMP). Manufacturers apply for an MRL, supplying the CVMP with two dossiers of information - on safety and residues - from which they can make their assessment.

The Safety Dossier contains all the pharmacology and toxicology studies carried out with the medicine in laboratory animals.

These studies examine what happens to the substance in the body and assess how much can be given safely, without inducing any unwanted adverse effects.

The safety dossier also includes the calculation of the ADI referred to earlier. This is based on results in laboratory animals and particularly on the so-called No-Observed-Effect Level (NOEL), the dose with no observable effect in the most sensitive test used.

The World Health Organisation recommends that once the NOEL has been determined, a safety factor of between 100 and 1000 (usually depending on the type of effect) is applied to derive the ADI.

The Residues Dossier contains all the data concerning the formation, nature, behaviour and disappearance of residues after a medicine has been given to a farm animal. Together, the results from the residues file on the quantities and behaviour of residues in farm animals, with the ADI derived from the safety file and the theoretical food intakes mentioned earlier (500 g meat, 1.5 litres of milk etc) are used to calculate the MRL(s), on the assumption that consumers get the maximum level every day of their lives.

Determining MRLs is a requirement of European legislation under a Council Regulation (2377/90). Under this legislation, substances must be entered into one of four annexes to the Regulation:

Annex I: Final MRLs

The data in the dossier are considered adequate to establish a final MRL.

Annex II: MRLs not Necessary

The data in the dossier demonstrate that there is no risk to the consumer and MRLs are not needed.

Annex III: Provisional MRLs

This is for medicines where MRLs can be established but some clarification of further studies are required before final MRLs can be set.

Annex IV

Residues of the medicine pose an unacceptable risk to the consumer or there is insufficient information to allow a full assessment. The products in Annex IV are prohibited for use in food producing animals in the European Union. No new medicine can be licensed or sold for use in food producing animals until its active ingredients have been entered into Annexes I, II or III of the Regulation.

Conclusion

Considerable research effort is put into developing the safety and residues dossiers for veterinary medicines so that the ADI values can be calculated, MRLs set and withdrawal periods established. This process, together with residues monitoring to ensure that residues above the MRL do not occur and that prohibited drugs are not used serves to ensure safety for the consumer, especially as large safety factors are built in at several stages of the process.

Violations of MRLs or the uses of prohibited substances, detected under the surveillance programme, are investigated and, where appropriate, are prosecuted. Legal sanctions can be taken against individuals who ignore instructions on the proper use of products.

Chapter 7

Animal Medicines

We know medicines help protect us from disease and can help get us better when we are ill, but there are a number of myths about the medicines given to keep the UK's farm animals healthy. Check out the following beliefs and challenge your assumptions

- Animals are given more vaccinations and medicines than are necessary or good for them
- Animal medicines are given to make money for farmers and vets
- You can't be sure that meat is safe to eat with all the vaccinations and medicines that animals are given now
- There are residues of animal medicines in our food
- Food from animals that have been vaccinated is not safe to eat
- Legislation around meat production and food safety is not tough enough
- Animals are given antibiotics to boost growth
- Animals are 'pumped up' with hormones to boost growth
- Animals are only given vaccinations and medicines because hygiene and living conditions standards are below par
- Animal medicines are only necessary in intensive farming
- Organically farmed animals are not given antibiotics
- Organic meat is healthier
- Organic farming is better for the environment
- Organic farming is more humane
- Animal medicines are a serious risk to human health.

Just as parents ensure their children are properly protected against disease, it is the responsibility of farmers to ensure the good health and well-being of the animals under their care. Vaccines are important in protecting animals from diseases that they are likely to encounter and may be difficult to treat. Other medicines are used to treat sick animals, or, for example, to protect them from parasite infestation.

The government, through the Veterinary Medicines Directorate (VMD), controls the quality, safety and effectiveness of the vaccines and medicines used in all animals.

The Veterinary Medicines Directorate, in conjunction with the Food Standards Agency and the Animal Health Agency, randomly collect samples from farm animals and from food of animal origin to ensure that it is safe to eat and that authorised medicines are being used both correctly and safely.

Animal medicines and vaccines help the farmer and vet ensure the good health and well-being of the animals under their care. They will be used as little as possible but as much as necessary

Animal medicines are given to make money for farmers and vets.

No. Animal medicines are used in farm animals, like pets and people, to prevent and control disease and illness. Animal medicines are just as sophisticated and effective as human medicines. They are expensive to produce and licence for use in farm animals.

The farmer and vet are responsible for the health and welfare of animals under their care. Medicines cost the farmer money – veterinary surgeons and other prescribers do not indiscriminately prescribe or supply medicines that are unnecessary for the health and welfare of animals. As well as prescribing medicines in response to a disease problem, veterinary surgeons and other advisers will often give farmers advice on the animal husbandry measures they can take to prevent a recurrence of disease.

You can't be sure that meat is safe to eat with all the vaccinations and medicines that animals are given now.

There is published information, from independent sources such as the Food Standards Agency and the Veterinary Residues Committee, readily available to show that meat and other food produced from animals is safe to eat.

The Veterinary Medicines Directorate (VMD) co-ordinates the collection of samples from foodstuffs such as meat, milk and eggs from both UK produce and imported produce. These food samples are analysed for residues derived from the use of veterinary medicines.

The VMD is responsible for the reporting of results. This work is overseen by the Veterinary Residues Committee, an independent advisory committee that oversees the UK's surveillance for residues of veterinary medicines. These results are published and readily available.

There are residues of animal medicines in our food.

Most animal food products do not contain any veterinary medicine residues.

In the event that food from animals does contain veterinary medicine residues, they will be at minute concentrations, below the 'no-effect level.'

The 'no-effect level' is the maximum dose of a substance that can be consumed over a stated period without producing detectable ill effects. The 'no effect level' is used to help calculate an appropriate 'withdrawal period' for the medicine. Until the withdrawal period has elapsed, the animal or its products must not be used for human consumption. The results of the veterinary medicines residues surveillance schemes which check that all is well are published by the Veterinary Medicines Directorate (VMD). They demonstrate that British farmers use medicines responsibly.

On the very rare occasions that unacceptable residues (residues above the maximum residue level) are found, the VMD works with the Food Standards Agency in a follow up investigation, and to instigate action to ensure public safety.

Food from animals that have been vaccinated is not safe to eat.

Vaccines work by stimulating the body to produce its own defence against infection. Mimicking what happens when an animal has been exposed to disease, the body and its defensive system will "remember" the identity of the invading organisms. Subsequent to this, if the animal comes into contact with the infectious disease agent (e.g. bacteria or virus) that the animal has been vaccinated against, its body is ready to fight it and the animal will not fall ill and suffer. This protects the individual animal and because of this the animal will not develop the disease and will not become infected.

A further benefit of vaccination is that where a significant proportion of the herd/flock is vaccinated, it helps protect the unvaccinated animals in that population from the disease, a concept known as "herd immunity".

Legislation around meat production and food safety is not tough enough.

Meat production and food safety are strictly regulated and controlled. British farmers and the animal health industry as well as those involved in processing food have to abide by strict controls. Their work is closely monitored and they are inspected regularly by government bodies including the Veterinary Medicines Directorate, the Animal Health Agency, Local Authority Environmental Health Officers and the Food Standards Agency. The work of the VMD is also overseen and monitored by the Veterinary Residues Committee, an independent advisory committee that manages the UK's surveillance programme for residues of veterinary medicines.

Recent consumer surveys show that there is public confidence in the established systems to ensure using medicines to protect farm animals' health and welfare will not adversely affect the safety of food from animals.

Animals are given antibiotics to boost growth.

Not true. At one time very small doses of some antibiotics were allowed to be added to feed because they improved the growth rates of some farm animals. But the EU phased out this practice, stopping the sale of antibiotic growth promoters on the 1st January 2006.

Animals are 'pumped up' with hormones to boost growth.

No – hormonal growth promoters have been banned since 1988 in the UK and the rest of the European Union.

Some hormones are used as medicines to treat sick cattle or to aid fertility control in cattle, pigs and sheep. They must only be prescribed under the strict control of a veterinarian. These products have been licensed as safe to use in food producing animals by the Veterinary Medicines Directorate, with withdrawal periods imposed to ensure no harmful residues can enter the food chain.

Animals are only given vaccinations and medicines because hygiene and living conditions standards are below par.

Animals, like people, need medicines too. Farmers use advice from professional veterinary surgeons, animal nutrition advisers and others to ensure that their livestock are kept healthy and their welfare is maintained in line with or better than the current animal welfare legislation.

Recent years have seen outbreaks of more "exotic" diseases such as Bluetongue, Avian Influenza and others and increasing levels of 'endemic' diseases such as Bovine Viral Diarrhoea and liver fluke. Such diseases are difficult to control and eradicate by good husbandry alone. Veterinary medicines, including vaccines, are tools that aid the good health and well-being of farm animals.

Animal medicines are only necessary in intensive farming.

Animals, like people, get ill and need medicines either to prevent or treat disease. Disease and illness occurs in all forms of farming. It is the duty of the farmer to ensure that the animals are healthy and husbandry practices comply with or exceed current animal health and welfare legislation.

Organically farmed animals are not given antibiotics.

Just as with people animals can be prescribed antibiotics to treat bacterial infections. If they were not then their welfare would suffer. This is the case in both organic and conventional systems of production.

Organic meat is healthier.

There is no evidence to suggest that organic meat is any healthier than conventionally produced meat. The balance of current scientific evidence does not support this view. Available evidence shows that the nutrient levels are similar in food produced by both organic and conventional agriculture.

Organic farming is better for the environment.

All types of farming require varying degrees of inputs to ensure the production of safe and nutritious food. Animals farmed under a variety of production systems are subject to disease and illness. Some researchers say that extensively produced organic food places a greater burden on the environment than efficiently grown conventional food as many more animals are needed to produce the same volume of food. Our land and resources are precious. With an expanding world population, more and more sophisticated methods of production will be required to feed the world. Organically produced food alone cannot meet the food (especially protein) demands that humanity requires.

Organic farming is more humane.

No, both organic and conventional food production in the UK must comply with current animal health, welfare and food hygiene legislation.

Animal medicines are a serious risk to human health.

Correctly used, animal medicines do not pose any risk to human health.

The animal medicines industry is committed to promoting responsible use of all types of medicines under the slogan 'as little as possible, as much as necessary'. By continuing to follow this principle when using medicines, farmers and veterinary surgeons can ensure that they remain available as a key tool to help maintain the health and welfare of the UK's farm animals.

Some Common Questions about Medicines for Farm Animals

Why do animals need veterinary medicines?

For Animal Welfare

We all have days when we feel fantastic, others when we are 'a bit under the weather' and times when, through no fault of our own, we are really quite poorly.

When we are ill most of us automatically turn to modern medicine to make us better. We can do this without a second thought because we know that the manufacturers have spent years developing their products to ensure their effectiveness and safety.

Ironically, the same people who would not hesitate to take medicine to ease their own pain or discomfort, sometimes believe that giving medicines to farm animals for the same reason is in some way wrong.

Like us, farm animals can also suffer from bacterial and viral diseases. In addition, like us, they can catch a cold, fall victim to a flu virus or suffer from what we might generally refer to as a 'stomach bug'. Whether housed indoors, even under the very best conditions, or kept outside, farm animals can suffer respiratory problems, or be affected by worms and external parasites such as lice and mites.

Unlike us, farm livestock can't communicate what is wrong with them. They rely on us to look after them and ensure they receive the medicines needed to treat the conditions that might cause distress or pain.

Many of us grow up with an image of healthy sheep and cattle grazing in the fields, chickens scratching in the yard or pigs rooting in the soil. One of the misconceptions is that livestock kept using extensive outdoor or organic systems are free from disease and infection. That is far from the case. Apart from the considerable risks sometimes posed by natural predators, animals kept under these conditions still have to contend with infections and parasitic diseases.

Farmers earn their living from the animals they keep, so it is in their interest to do everything they can to look after their livestock. Farmers go to great lengths to select the right breed of animal for their specific farm conditions and end markets. They also take care to ensure that the animals are housed to high standards and fed the right diet to ensure they grow up healthy and strong.

Prevention of Disease

To help maintain farm animals in the condition most people would like to see, farmers sometimes have to use modern medicines, which are more advanced, safer and effective than ever before. Where suitable products exist, the best way to ensure good health is often to prevent infection taking hold in the first place. In exactly the same way that we might have our children vaccinated when they are young, to avoid major difficulties later in life, medicines, such as vaccines are used to prevent potential health problems in our farm animals. Veterinary surgeons work closely with farmers to develop preventative programmes designed to maintain the health of their animals or birds.

Treatment of Disease

Because preventative treatments are used to ensure their welfare, most farm animals remain healthy throughout their lives. However, where effective preventative treatments are not available, remedial treatments, such as antibiotics, might be used to help get them back on their feet, to prevent others members of the herd or flock from being infected, or to prevent unhealthy animals from entering the human food chain.

For Healthy Food

The explosion in the world's population means that during the next 30 years farmers will have to produce as much food as they have done in the whole of the last 10,000 years. That will be a huge task when, even today, many of the world's population do not receive an adequate diet. The use of modern medicines to ensure the animals we farm remain healthy and productive will play a major role in achieving that aim.

Let's look at the reasons why.

Healthy food comes from healthy animals, so it makes sense to ensure farm livestock are always in the best possible health. Healthy animals grow more quickly, make the best use of the food they eat and produce good quality foodstuffs, such as meat, dairy products and eggs, at affordable prices. They also provide us with essential by-products such as wool and leather.

In contrast, sick or suffering animals not only cost more to feed but because diseases may affect the eating or keeping quality of what they produce, the meat, milk or eggs they produce often cannot be sold. In more extreme cases, it may even be unsafe to eat food from animals that could be carrying disease.

Medicines are essential if these hazards are to be effectively controlled. In fact, one of the requirements for eggs to qualify for the recognised 'Lion' quality mark for eggs is that the chickens that produce them are vaccinated against salmonella.

Professional livestock farmers earn their living from the animals they keep, so naturally it is in their interest to do everything they can to look after their livestock. Farmers are careful to select the right breed of animal for their specific farm conditions, take care that the animals are housed to high standards and that they are fed the right diet so they grow healthy and strong.

In the UK, farmers and veterinarians have an excellent track record of using animal medicines safely and responsibly to help achieve these aims. Every time a farm animal is treated, a record must be kept. Furthermore, the animal or its produce (eggs or milk) may not enter the food chain until a specified period (the 'withdrawal' period) following medication has passed.

The use of modern medicines is essential now and will become even more important in the future if our farmers are to meet the world's food needs.

How do we know that the medicines used are safe?

Although some people worry about farm animals being given medicines, the majority of us realise that there is little cause for concern, and many good reasons why we should use them.

Animal medicine companies invest huge resources in developing, testing and manufacturing safe, effective medicines. Without them, veterinary surgeons and farmers would be unable to carry out their job properly and look after the welfare of our farm animals. Just think how you would feel if you went to your local GP and found the surgery had no modern-day treatments!

It should be reassuring to know that Europe has one of the world's most stringent licensing systems for controlling veterinary medicines. In the UK, the Veterinary Medicines Directorate (VMD), an executive agency of the Department for Environment, Food & Rural Affairs (DEFRA), is responsible for authorising and controlling the manufacture and marketing of animal medicines. To protect consumers, it also carries out checks to make sure there are no harmful residues of animal medicines present in meat and other animal products.

To ensure that animal medicines reaching the market are safe to use and effective, manufacturers have to operate within a strict regulatory framework, according to very strict scientific criteria. This ensures that the medicines we use are of good quality, do what they are supposed to do and are safe to livestock, to the people that administer them, to the environment and ultimately, for farm animals, to the consumers of any produce for these animals.

Why do some medicines have to be prescribed by vets?

We have already talked about how most of us instinctively reach for the aspirin when we get a headache. Like many other low-dose general medicines, aspirin is easily available over the counter and comes with easy-to-follow instructions telling us how much to take. There are also other medicines which can't be bought from the supermarket, but which can be brought from a pharmacy without going to the doctor for a prescription. Similarly, many routine animal health medicines can be prescribed to farmers by pharmacists, or suitably qualified persons at animal health merchants operating under a Code of Practice. These trained staff qualified to give advice on responsible use. These products carry full instructions, approved by the VMD, on how to use the product.

Many of the more potent drugs and treatments that keep humans healthy are only available on prescription after a proper consultation with a trained GP. Similarly, there are times when only a POM-V (Prescription Only Medicine - Veterinary) will do when it comes to treating animals. Only veterinary surgeons can prescribe POM-Vs for animals under their care, which is what you would expect. It is the job of the veterinary surgeon to correctly diagnose what is wrong, then prescribe and sometimes administer the most appropriate treatment correctly and safely. This ensures the well-being and safety of the animal being treated and, ultimately, the consumer.

For the same reasons that pharmaceutical companies are continually developing new medicines to treat human ailments, so too it is important that veterinary surgeons and farmers are able to choose from a wide range of modern, safe and effective animal medicines. Some medicines, such as new generation vaccines or oral rehydration solutions are even leading the way for human medicine development.

In no small part, the quality, safety and relatively low cost of the food products we now enjoy is due to the extensive research invested by the animal health industry in products to ensure the health of our farm livestock.

Pharmacovigilance: Monitoring Suspected Adverse Reactions to Animal Medicines

Introduction

Thankfully, harmful, unexpected side-effects to animal medicines are extremely uncommon. Before any animal medicine is allowed onto the UK market it has, by law, to satisfy very strict criteria on its quality, its effectiveness and its safety. However, once an animal medicine is in use, it is vital to know if any animals or people suffer unexpected problems following use or exposure to the product under field conditions.

Very occasionally animals may show some small mild reaction to a medicine - just as you may feel drowsy after certain common medications. But, if your animal is unwell after treatment with an animal medicine or if you are at all worried, contact your vet. This is just common-sense, whether or not your animal has received medication, and it is more than likely that the illness is totally unrelated to the medicine.

Suspected Adverse Reaction Surveillance Scheme

The Veterinary Medicines Directorate (VMD), which administers the licensing system, runs a scheme to monitor reports of any reactions in animals, people or the environment following the use of animal medicines, called the Suspected Adverse Reaction Surveillance Scheme.

The purpose of the scheme is to monitor trends in reported suspected reactions. Reports received by the VMD are prioritised in terms of severity and likely causality (i.e. to see whether the problem is likely to be linked to the medicine). The scheme also analyses whether there have been any other reports about the same product or others like it, whether any further information is required and whether any follow-up is required.

The Legal Background

Title VII of the Veterinary Medicinal Products Directive 2001/82/EC, headed Pharmacovigilance, imposes certain duties on holders of marketing authorisations. The European Committee for Veterinary Medicinal Products adopted a Note for Guidance entitled *Pharmacovigilance of Veterinary Medicinal Products* which came into operation on 1 January 1998.

This European guideline sets out the recommended framework for pharmacovigilance which places specific duties on conditions attached to individual product authorisations. Duties are also placed on member states' competent authorities (the VMD in the UK).

Company Responsibilities

Article 74 of Directive 2001/82/EC requires the holder of each marketing authorisation to "have permanently and continuously at his disposal an appropriately qualified person responsible for pharmacovigilance".

The appropriately qualified person is responsible for setting up and operating a system which ensures that all information about any suspected adverse reactions reported to the company is collected and collated at a single point. Records of suspected adverse reactions must by law be kept for at least 5 years.

Periodic Safety Update reports should be sent in on the request of the Suspected Adverse Reaction Surveillance Scheme or as required by the VMD. Generally, however, they are submitted six-monthly for the first 2 years after product authorisation, annually for the subsequent 3 years, and thereafter every 5 years.

This report lists all the suspected adverse reactions reported to the company since the last Periodic Safety Update report. This is set into context by looking at the incidence of reactions, taking account of the number of doses sold. Each Periodic Safety Update report should contain a concise assessment of the evaluation of the current safety of the product.

Reporting Suspected Adverse Reactions

If an adverse reaction to an animal medicine is suspected, it should be reported to the scheme and/or the company involved. Your vet or doctor will normally do this: they are actively encouraged to do so by both the VMD and NOAH, but the VMD welcomes anyone reporting such adverse reactions they have experienced or observed. Yellow forms for doing this are available from the VMD.

Often, vets will contact the manufacturer directly to report a suspected adverse reaction. Companies are then under a legal obligation to report these to the VMD - half of all reports come directly from companies.

Only by professionals and owners taking the trouble to report any problems can the VMD and companies get an idea of any action that may need to be taken. This could ultimately mean withdrawing the product or a specific batch from the market, but more usually it will result in more advice being given to users of the medicine as to how to use it safely, or on possible side-effects. NOAH encourages active reporting of suspected adverse reactions, but is pleased that there are so few. This shows that the authorisation system for animal medicines is doing its job and protecting animals and the public from potential danger.

Definitions

Adverse reaction: a reaction which is harmful and unintended and which occurs at doses normally used in animals for the prophylaxis, diagnosis or treatment of disease or the modification of physiological function (Article 1(10) of Directive 2001/82/EC).

Human Adverse Reaction: an incident where a person reports adverse effects following exposure to a veterinary medicinal product.

Suspected adverse reaction (SAR): any report indicating that there has or may have been an adverse reaction to a product. The Suspected Adverse Reaction Surveillance Scheme treats all reports of adverse reactions as suspected until shown to be otherwise.

Poultry Medicines

Why use Poultry Medicines?

Poultry, like humans, can suffer from infectious disease. Birds deserve the protection of modern medicines.

What are Poultry Medicines?

Just as in humans, poultry medicines are used to prevent and cure disease. They fall into two categories; vaccines and pharmaceuticals. Because of the need to prevent disease spreading, it is usual to treat all the birds in a house or pen at the same time.

Vaccines

Vaccines are preventive medicines which stimulate the body's natural immune system to protect against a particular disease or parasite.

Poultry vaccines, like human vaccines, can be either live or inactivated.

(i)   Live vaccines - usually given in the drinking water, or by aerosol spray or injection. These help protect birds of all ages.

(ii) Inactivated vaccines - given by injection, usually to older birds before the start of egg production, to protect both the bird and its offspring.

Pharmaceuticals

Pharmaceuticals (antibiotics or synthetic chemicals) are given in water or feed. Water-based products are generally used to treat outbreaks of parasitic or bacterial diseases; in-feed products may be used either for prevention or treatment.

How are Medicines Approved?

In the UK, all medicines for animal use must be licensed under the Medicines Act 1968, various EC Directives and Regulations and their subsequent Statutory Instruments. This involves thorough examination by independent scientific experts and officials on behalf of the Licensing Authority.

To obtain a marketing authorisation, formerly called a "product licence", a company has to provide a great deal of information about the product. It must carry out extensive scientific tests to prove it can meet very strict standards on safety, quality and effectiveness. The dossier containing the results of these tests must be sent to the Veterinary Medicines Directorate of DEFRA, or for a product going for EU-wide approval, to the European Medicines Evaluation Agency.

Every batch of the product has to reach high quality standards demanded by the experts and show that a quality control programme has been established to ensure this. The company must also show, through clinical trials, that the product will do what they say it will do - that it is effective.

But above all, the company must show that the product is safe: safe not only for the bird which receives it, but safe for the human who consumes the poultry meat or eggs produced from the bird, safe for the farmer who administers the medicine, safe for the environment, and, if the medicine is incorporated in feed, safe for the mill worker who prepares the feed.

Extensive tests are also performed to make sure that no harmful residues of the medicine remain in the poultry meat, or eggs. A withdrawal period is approved for each product calculated on the basis of its Maximum Residue Limit (MRL). The bird cannot be used for human consumption, neither can any eggs be sold, until this period has passed.

To protect the environment, the company must also prove that the use of the medicine will not harm wildlife, fish or plants, or cause river or soil pollution. Only when the Licensing Authority is satisfied, is the product authorised for use.

Poultry medicine labels carry detailed information and the product data sheet gives even more. The information includes how the medicine can be used, the dosage, method of administration, contra-indications, how long before the bird or its eggs enter the food chain must the medicine be withdrawn from use, and how the medicine must be stored. All this must be agreed as part of the authorisation process.

Why are Poultry Medicines Approved?

It is essential to ensure that users of the products and consumers of poultry meat or eggs can have confidence in what they use and eat.

The licensing system is the background to that confidence.

What other Safeguards are There?

The sale and supply of animal medicines in the UK is strictly controlled by the Veterinary Medicines Directorate and policed by the Royal Pharmaceutical Society of Great Britain. Depending on their classification, licensed poultry medicines may only be purchased from a veterinary surgeon, pharmacist or registered animal health distributor.

Poultry vaccines are classified as either 'Pharmacy and Merchants List' (PML) and available from registered merchants, or 'Prescription Only Medicine' (POM) which are available only on the prescription of a vet.

Products to be incorporated in feed are mostly classified MFS, which means they may only be included in the feed in accordance with an MFS Prescription from a vet (formerly Veterinary Written Direction). A number of in-feed products are classified as MFSX, which means they are exempt from the need for a prescription.

As described above, all medicines come with detailed manufacturers' instructions on how to use them. In addition, for antibiotics, there is additional advice, such as the RUMA Guidelines for the Responsible Use of Antibiotics for Poultry. Young birds are more susceptible to some diseases, so medicines may only need to be given at the start of a bird's life. Scrupulous records of all medicine use must be kept by farmers, showing the date and details of treatment, plus a note of any required withdrawal period before birds may be slaughtered or their products, such as eggs, may enter the food chain. This helps with traceability.

All birds intended for human consumption are examined by slaughterhouse inspectors for evidence of disease or injury and, under the terms of the Statutory Surveillance Scheme, random samples of poultry meat (labelled with the farm of origin) are taken for residue testing to ensure that producers have adhered to the rules.

Conclusion

Medicines are essential for animal welfare and healthy, reasonably priced food. Use of licensed medicines provides assurances of quality, performance and safety to farmers and consumers.

Veterinary Medicines Regulations

The Veterinary Medicinal Products Directive 2001/82/EC (as amended) sets out the controls on the manufacture, authorisation, marketing, distribution and post-authorisation surveillance of veterinary medicines applicable in all European Member States. The Directive provides the basis for the UK controls on veterinary medicines, which are set out nationally in the Veterinary Medicines Regulation. The Regulations are revoked and replaced on an annual basis after consultation with interested groups to ensure that they are up-to-date and fit for purpose.

Veterinary Medicines Regulations 2011 SI 2159 (VMR) and Veterinary Medicines Guidance Notes (VMGN):

The Veterinary Medicines Regulations 2011 (SI 2159) (VMR) came into force on 1 October 2011.

The VMR first came into force in October 2005 to implement Directive 2001/82 and consolidate all the controls on veterinary medicines that were previously part of the Medicines Act 1968 and over 50 amending Statutory Instruments. The VMR also implement EU legislation relating to medicated feeds, and some specified feed additives used in feeding stuffs.

The VMR are regularly updated and some of the key changes they introduce this time are:

- a waiver for fees for variations to marketing authorisations seeking to remove or reduce animal tests;
- simplification of the procedure for dealing with variations to national marketing authorisations;
- a revision of the exemptions concerning animals kept on domestic premises, to remove the ceiling on weight of medicated feeding stuff that can be manufactured from premixtures;
- a derogation allowing veterinary surgeons and pharmacists to supply premixtures and medicated feed intended for domestic use without the need to be approved as a distributor;

- a procedure and a fee for applications for advice as to whether or not a product requires a marketing authorisation.

Hard copies may be purchased from the Stationary Office (TSO).

The Impact Assessment (142 kb) for the VMR provides information on the decision making process.

The Veterinary Medicines Guidance Notes, which accompany the VMR, have also been revised by the VMD to reflect the legislative changes and to comply with the Anderson review on guidance. The Anderson review aimed to improve the regulatory guidance that the government gives to business.

The VMD guidance notes provide professionals working in the veterinary sector with clear information on different aspects of the legislation on veterinary medicines.

On the Responsible Use pf Animal Medicinss

Introduction

Animal medicines play an important role in the control and prevention of disease and animal suffering but have the potential to cause harm if not used properly. In the UK, consumers have long enjoyed the benefits of rigorous systems designed to protect them from harmful residues of such medicines in their food. These include statutory controls on the authorisation, distribution and use of such medicines.

Authorisation of Animal Medicines

The VMD is responsible for the authorisation and control of the manufacture and marketing of animal medicines and for surveillance for residues of animal medicines in meat and other animal products.

Diagnosis and Prevention of Disease

Veterinary surgeons ensure that animal diseases are properly diagnosed and can help to design preventive programmes such as Flock/Herd or Animal Health Plans. You should therefore consult your veterinary surgeon when a diagnosis of disease and treatment for your animals may be needed or when you need to design or modify a preventive disease programme.

Distribution Categories of Animal Medicines

Once a disease has been diagnosed and treatment prescribed or a preventive programme designed, it may be necessary to obtain an animal medicine. All animal medicines in the UK are assigned into one of four distribution categories:

Prescription Only Medicines - Veterinarian (POM-V)

A veterinary medicinal product classified as a POM-V may only be supplied once it has been prescribed by a veterinary surgeon following a clinical assessment of the animal (or group of animals) which must be under the care of the prescribing veterinarian. This category includes veterinary medicines that were previously classified as MFS. POM-V products may only be supplied by veterinary surgeons and pharmacists.

Prescription Only Medicines – Veterinarian, Pharmacist, Suitably Qualified Person (SPQ) (POM-VPS)

A veterinary medicinal product classified as POM-VPS may only be prescribed by either a registered veterinary surgeon, pharmacist or Suitably Qualified Person (SQP). An SQP is a person who is trained and registered to be able to sell a limited range of veterinary products and often works from a pet shop, saddlery or agricultural merchant's premises. A clinical assessment of the animal(s) is not a prerequisite when prescribing this category of veterinary medicines and the animal does not have to be under the care of a veterinarian. The person prescribing, however, must be satisfied that the person administering the medicine has the competence to do so safely and that the medicine is intended for its authorised use. The prescriber must provide advice on how to use the product, making specific reference to any warnings or contra-indications relevant to the medicine.

Non-Food Animal – Veterinarian, Pharmacist, SQP (NFA-VPS)

A veterinary medicinal product classified as NFA-VPS may only be supplied by either a registered veterinary surgeon, pharmacist or SQP. As with POM-VPS medicines, a clinical assessment of the animal(s) is not a prerequisite for supply of this category. The supplier, however, must be satisfied that the person administering the medicine has the competence to do so safely and the medicine is intended for its authorised use. The supplier must also provide advice related to any warnings or contra-indications relevant to it and also advise on how the product has to be administered.

Authorised Veterinary Medicine – General Sales List (AVM-GSL)

A veterinary medicinal product classified as an AVM-GSL may be supplied by any retailer as there are no restrictions on its supply.

Safe Use of Animal Medicines on Farm

Ultimately it is the farmer who is responsible for ensuring that animal medicines are used in a safe, responsible and effective way in accordance with a prescription. The following Code of Practice has been drawn up to provide you with guidelines to help you to fulfil this responsibility. *This Code is intended as a general guide and should not be treated as a complete or authoritative statement of the law on any particular case.*

Plan Ahead to Prevent Disease

1. *Prevention is the best policy.* Draw up a clear Animal Health Plan. It would be useful to work with your veterinary surgeon to identify the best ways to prevent or treat disease in your animals and to ensure their welfare is fully taken into account, including any necessary changes in farm practice. Ensure that your plan includes all the medicines you are using including those incorporated in medicated feeding stuffs.

2. *Consult your veterinary surgeon* when you require the diagnosis of any animal health problem and advice on the most appropriate animal medicines available to treat or prevent disease. A pharmacist or SQP can provide information on the medicines that they can lawfully supply. However, they are not qualified to carry out a clinical assessment of the animals.

Development of Non-antibiotic Tactics to Control Mastitis

Mastitis will cost Michigan dairy producers approximately $50 million in lost revenues annually. Some obvious costs associated with mastitis control include medications, labour, and veterinary services. However, most of the economic losses due to mastitis are attributed to reduced milk production, discarded antibiotic-treated milk, and increased need for replacement animals.

Over the past several decades, procedures that improve milking time hygiene and reduce the exposure of udders to infectious pathogens have proven to be highly effective in reducing the incidence of some forms of mastitis. For example, prevalence of contagious pathogens such as Staphylococcus aureus and Streptococcus agalactiae has decreased considerably with the application of these good management practices. Unfortunately, the etiology (cause or origin) of mastitis has shifted over the years from contagious organisms to more environmental pathogens, even in well-managed herds. The environmental pathogens, such as Escherichia coli and Klebsiella pneumoniae, are often associated with more frequent episodes of clinical mastitis that can pose some unique challenges for eliminating existing intramammary infections (1).

Antibiotic therapy as a means to treat infections is an important part of current mastitis control programs. Historically, formulations of both lactating and dry-cow intramammary products were directed primarily against the gram-positive organisms, particularly staphylococci and streptococci. Indeed, most over-the-counter infusion products are highly effective in treating many forms of streptococcal mastitis.

However, the therapeutic success rates with antibiotic therapy can vary considerably depending on the duration of infection and the specific organisms causing the infection. Chronic Staph, aureus mastitis has proven to be very difficult to eliminate during lactation using currently available intramammary treatment products due to buildup of scar tissue and abscess formation. In recent years, there also has been an emergence of mastitis-causing pathogens that have a greater resistance to antibiotic therapies, including coliforms and Mycoplasma bovis (2).

Despite the dire economic impact of this disease on the dairy industry, the most widely accepted method of mastitis therapy remains intramammary antibiotic treatment. In reality, the efficacy (effectiveness) of such treatments is low during the lactation period, especially against major mastitis-causing pathogens. This method of treatment is not always cost-effective either due to discarded antibiotic-contaminated milk during and after treatment. Estimates suggest that antibiotic contaminated milk will cost the US dairy industry $50 million annually. Antibiotic residues are an undesirable consequence of controlling mastitis, and there is a growing concern from consumers over the potential presence of drug residues in the food supply.

In a survey conducted by the National Dairy Board, consumers listed antibiotics as a serious health hazard in the food supply. When questioned about milk, the majority of the respondents listed chemical residues as a problem and wanted the Federal government to increase antibiotic regulation to ensure food safety (3). While the vast majority of dairy farmers use antibiotics in a responsible fashion, there are some groups who blame antibiotic usage on dairy farms for the emergence of antibiotic resistant human pathogens. It is obvious that new approaches are needed to reduce the dairy industry's dependence on chemotherapy as its major means for reducing or eliminating existing intramammary infections.

Non-antiobiotic Approaches

It is well established that the changes in incidence and severity of mastitis are related directly to changes in the composition, magnitude, and efficiency of the udder's immune system. In order to address the future needs of the dairy industry, researchers are investigating ways to enhance the natural defence mechanisms of the udder to prevent and effectively eliminate mastitis.

For example, certain immune cells (lymphocytes) in the cow's udder are capable of secreting natural antibacterial proteins that can kill a spectrum of common mastitis-causing bacteria including coliforms, Strep uberis, and Staph aureu. Initial safety studies showed that this antibacterial protein does not adversely affect the udder, but still has potent activity against bacteria present in the milk.

Further characterisation of this antibacterial protein suggested that it may belong to a family of proteins that also are found in human lymphocytes called saposin-like proteins (SAPLIP). Indeed, through the use of gene databases and molecular techniques it was confirmed that a bovine homologue of SAPLIP exists in udder lymphocytes that is very similar in structure and function with human SAPLIP. Studies currently are underway at MSU's College of Veterinary Medicine to purify large quantities of the bovine SAPLIP in order to explore ways that it could be used to control bacterial infections in dairy cattle.

It is possible that this factor could be used as a natural antimicrobial agent for the therapeutic treatment of mastitis-causing pathogens. Bovine SAPLIP also may be useful in teat dip formulations for both the pre- and post-milking applications. The successful development of this new technology may have several advantages over conventional chemotherapies in eliminating mastitis, including:

1. a broad spectrum of activity to kill different bacterial species (Staph. aureus, *E. coli*, streptococci) without causing damage to host cells;

2. minimal contribution to the emerging resistance of bacterial pathogens to antibacterial drugs; and,

3. the elimination of undesirable residues from contaminating animal products destined for human consumption.

Results from these studies may lead to development of new strategies to control mastitis and provide a viable alternative to less effective mastitis control procedures based on traditional chemotherapy.

Footrot in Cattle

It is an infection of the soft tissue between the claws (digits) of the feet and is caused by two anaerobic bacteria (these are bacteria that grow in the absence of oxygen), Fusobacterium necrophorum and Bacteroides melaninogenicus. These bacteria are common in the environment and F. necrophorum is present in the rumen and feces of normal cattle. Fusobacterium necrophorum is the same agent that causes liver abscesses in dairy cattle and feedlot calves. Once these bacteria invade the skin of the foot, they rapidly cause the condition we recognise as footrot. Injury or damage to the skin between the claws allows this invasion to occur.

Common factors that can cause damage of this sort include stubble fields, small rocks and pebbles, and abrasive surfaces. Additionally, high temperatures and excess moisture or humidity causes the skin between the claws to chap and crack allowing these bacteria to invade. The wet spring this year, the lush pastures in many areas, and the advent of hot weather may provide the ideal conditions for footrot to become a major problem this summer.

The appearance of footrot is fairly typical and begins as a swelling of the skin between the claws. This swelling usually occurs within 24 hours of the onset of the infection. The toes become separated due to the swelling and the skin appears reddened. The foot is very painful and the animal can be quite lame at this time. A fissure or crack develops along the swollen area for part or all of the length of the space between the toes (the interdigital space). Yellow to grayish tissue extends from this crack and the lesion has a characteristic foul odour. The British call this disease "foul of foot" which is very descriptive. The area around the coronary band can be swollen and red. Affected cattle can have a mild fever, refuse feed, and be mildly to severely lame. Also, it is common for affected cattle to lose a considerable amount of weight during a bout of footrot. If the footrot lesion does not heal satisfactorily, very serious problems can develop. The structures just beneath the skin of the foot include the bones of the foot, the tendons and joints of the foot. If these underlying structures are invaded by bacteria-particularly the joints, bones, or tendons—therapy is very difficult and the chances of recovery are low.

Footrot can usually be recognised in typical cases; however, a number of conditions can be confused with footrot. These conditions include corns, puncture wounds due to nails, needles, or other sharp objects, sole abscesses, fractures of the bones of the foot, and a newly recognised condition that primarily affects dairy cattle, "hairy foot warts." All lame feet should be carefully examined and it should not be assumed that all lame cattle have footrot. If you have any questions regarding lameness problems affecting your cattle, you should contact your veterinarian for diagnosis and advice.

Treatment of footrot is relatively straightforward and if instituted early is usually successful. For mild cases, local treatment can be accomplished by thoroughly cleaning the foot, and then applying an astringent (such as 5% copper sulfate). For moderate or severe cases, systemic antibiotic therapy is usually recommended. Antibiotics that are usually effective include penicillin, oxytetracycline, ampicillin, or sulfa drugs. All label directions should be carefully followed including withdrawal times before slaughter.

If a dose higher than that listed on the label is used, the antibiotic is being used in an extralabel manner and a veterinarian's prescription is needed and an extended withdrawal time determined by your veterinarian must be observed. Also, if the drug is not approved for treatment of footrot, a prescription is needed. If the animal does not improve (with noticeably less lameness) within a day or two or if deeper structures of the foot become infected, consult your veterinarian immediately.

One preventive measure is to insure that damage to the feet of cattle is minimised. This includes making sure cattle do not have to be in muddy areas for extended periods of time. Limiting coarse stubble grazing to cooler times of the year and limiting contact with gravelly or rocky areas. Some of these problems may not be avoidable under practical conditions. Other preventive measures that have been recommended include footbaths, feeding of organic iodine, feeding of zinc methionine, and/or vaccines.

Footbaths can be used to prevent cases; however, they are not particularly useful in the face of an outbreak. The common footbath solutions are (1) 2% formalin, and (2) 5% copper sulfate. Both compounds must be used with extreme caution from both animal health and environmental aspects. In fact, formalin solutions are very caustic and will damage your skin or eyes if splashed or spilled and are not generally recommended except in the face of extreme problems. Copper sulfate can be fatal to cattle if they drink it and must be disposed of carefully to avoid damaging aquatic plants or animals. Footbaths should be used 3 times per week to be effective and should not be used for long periods of time (greater than 3 weeks). The cattle should have clean feet before entering the foot baths (pre-washing may be necessary) and only about 300 head can be done before the solution should be changed. Feeding organic iodine (ethylenediamine dihydriodide; EDDI) can help prevent footrot. The EDDI should be fed at 10-15 milligrams per head per day. Feeding more than this will not be any more effective and can cause the cattle to have excess salivation. EDDI fed in loose salt mixes works very well. EDDI should not be fed in salt block formulations as it does not seem to be available to the cattle. Zinc methionine (Zinpro®) is also thought to be helpful in preventing footrot in feedlot situations and might be of value in range or pasture situations.

There are commercial vaccines that have limited effectiveness in preventing footrot in cattle; it is important to strategically administer these vaccines so that maximum protection is achieved during the time of year when cattle are most at risk (summer). Your veterinarian will also know of local factors that may be important in preventing footrot, so be sure to discuss this matter with him/her before spending a lot of time, money or effort on control and prevention measures. Since footrot is an infectious disease it is important that your cattle's immunity is normal and thus a good feeding and supplementation program is necessary.

We see many more footrot problems in beef herds that are copper deficient or selenium deficient. So make sure your cattle are not short on either of these trace minerals. The key to managing footrot is prevention, because treating a large number of individual animals can take a lot of the fun out of summer.

Chapter 8

Respiratory Disease in Young Dairy Calves

Respiratory problems have increased by 34 per cent in the last 20 years, causing nearly 21 per cent of all newborn calf losses. Heifers that survive continue to perform poorly as adult cows. In order to prevent this costly problem, it is important to address both determinant and predisposing causes.

Predisposing Causes

Passive Immunity – To be able to survive the microbial challenges posed immediately after birth, a calf must have built-up adequate immunity. As there is little time to develop its own immune system, the calf needs to rely on the passive immunity received from the dam through colostrum.

To guarantee that colostrum feeding transfers passive immunity, the four key attributes of colostrum feeding—quality, quantity, quickness, and cleanliness—must be observed.

Current guidelines suggest calves should receive 3–4 quarts of high-quality colostrum within 1 hour of birth and 3 additional quarts in 12 hours. If colostrum ingestion is inadequate, esophageal feeders can be used making sure that 3–4 quarts are administered within 1 hour of birth. The majority of the dairies in the US feed colostrum to calves from either a bucket or a bottle. Pooling colostrum is also becoming popular with these farms because it increases the immune competence of the calves (or their ability to respond to a more diverse pool of pathogens). When pooling colostrum, care must be taken to ensure not to include colostrum either from cows having Johnes or from 1st calf heifers.

One way to find out if colostrum has supplied adequate amounts of immunoglobulins (IgG) is to measure either IgG directly or serum total protein in blood serum. Serum total protein measured with a refractometre is highly correlated with serum IgG levels. Measuring serum total protein in a group of calves is more meaningful than individual readings. At least 80 per cent of a group of calves should have serum protein levels of 5.5 g/dL or higher.

While timely colostrum administration is critical, so is proper handling, as colostrum can be an ideal growth medium for bacteria. If colostrum is not going to be fed immediately, it is very important to refrigerate or freeze the colostrum as soon as possible. A recent study of Minnesota and Wisconsin dairies has shown that the mean total bacteria count and total coliform count in over 200 colostrum samples collected was 16.1 million and 2.7 million cfu/ml, respectively. Thus, the first approach should be to collect colostrum under strict sanitary conditions and cool the colostrum as soon as possible.

Some producers are evaluating the possibility of on-farm pasteurisation to make colostrum safer. Research trials have shown no difference in colostral IgG concentration between raw and pasteurised colostrum. What's really important though is that the trials have also shown a reduction in the mean total bacteria counts at time of feeding (813 and 40,738 cfu/ml for pasteurised and raw colostrum, respectively. In addition, calves fed pasteurised colostrum had higher IgG levels in blood (22.34 mg/ml and 18.07 mg/ml for pasteurised and raw colostrum, respectively).

If pasteurisation is going to be used, a batch pasteuriser is recommended, as it uses relatively lower temperatures and a longer heating time (60°C for 60-120 minutes) without risking denaturing the immunoglobulins and thus reducing colostrum quality. Due to the cost of the equipment, this alternative is mostly reserved for large dairy operations that have to feed greater numbers of newborn calves at one time. Needless to say, milk pasteurisers can also be used for waste milk, which reduces the costs of using milk replacers.

Environment — Raising calves in barns is convenient because it protects the calves and the employees from adverse weather. The problem is that stationary, warm air can contain potentially harmful gases (i.e., ammonia), odour, dust, and microorganisms (e.g., fungal spores, viruses, and bacteria). Ammonia and dust can reach the alveoli of the calf's lung and cause irritation and inflammatory reactions. Dust particles oftentimes carry microbes that can reach respiratory tissues where they can multiply. This association between respiratory diseases and air quality in confinement environments has been recognised for a long time.

Other factors that increase the risk of respiratory disease are shared housing with cows during the first week of life, more than 2 months difference in age within a group, previous episodes of diarrhea compared with none, and leaving calves with dams for more than 24 hours post calving. Maintaining clean-and-dry quarters for all calves is of utmost importance to reduce the incidence of respiratory disease.

To reduce bacterial numbers in the environment, important management measures, such as increasing pen area and decreasing pen temperature, can be taken (table 1). Increasing pen area results in less microbe concentration per surface unit and thus less challenge for the calves. Cold-temperature housing has also beneficial effects, as bacterial growth is reduced under cold conditions. A recent experiment compared calf performance under cold (40.5°F) and warm (59.9°F) indoor environment. Calves were fed 1 pound per day of a non-medicated milk replacer that contained 20 percent protein and 20 percent fat. Environmental temperature had no effect on scour scores, days scouring, and electrolyte costs. Calves subjected to cold conditions consumed more grain starter, which resulted in similar growth rates between both environments.

This demonstrates that calves need additional nutrients when cold-temperature barns are used. The performance success of calves in cold housing thus depends on administering adequate nutrition.

Adequate ventilation is critical to reduce not only bacteria counts in the air but also ammonia concentration, which irritates the respiratory tract. However, producers have to be able to differentiate between proper ventilation and drafts that result in cold stress. In a recent experiment, the absence of drafts was associated with reduced risk for diarrhea and respiratory disease.

A calf that is in its thermoneutral zone will not resort to energy-production or energy-saving mechanisms to cope with cold stress. Producers can check the calves to verify that cold-coping strategies such as shivering or pilo-erection (hair rising) have not been set in motion by the body. Checking the depth of the hair coat in calves is a good, practical way of assessing mild cold stress that has not elicited shivering. At environmental temperatures of 73°F, the depth of the coat can be nearly half an inch, whereas when pilo-erection occurs in response to cold the depth of the coat will almost double.

To cope with cold weather, calves need adequate nutrition and dry, well-insulated surface to rest on. Characteristics desired in bedding sources for calves are good moisture absorbance and the ability to keep the body warm. One study found that wheat straw had the warmest surface temperature, rice hulls and wood shavings had intermediate temperature, and sand had the lowest temperature. The concentration of ammonia at 4 inches above the bedding was also lowest for long wheat straw. Another study also found wheat straw to be warmer, and although it supported greater bacterial counts than wood products (i.e., shavings or sawdust), it appeared the bacterial problem was overcome by the straw improving calf nesting and thus environmental temperature control.

Determinant Cause: Microorganisms

Assuming calves have received adequate immunity through colostrum, the next important step it to reduce the microbial challenge. In order to accomplish this, the calf has to be removed from the dam as soon as possible. Calves should be placed in their own quarters in individual pens that help them avoid nose-to-nose contact with other calves. This environment should help the calves cope with stress by reducing exposure to pathogens from the cow and other calves. There should be ample dry bedding that will provide comfort and insulation from the cold. Be sure to avoid bedding materials that will result in dust (e.g., sawdust), as dust irritates the respiratory tract and facilitates the attack by bacteria.

Numerous vaccines are marketed for prevention of clinical respiratory diseases in cattle. Traditional views have held that the antibodies the calf receives through colostrum usually cause vaccines given to a young calf to be ineffective. More recent research indicates that, in certain instances, modified live viral vaccines stimulate a protective response in calves challenged with these agents, despite the inability to measure an active antibody response in the calf's bloodstream. An example of this protection is the use of intranasal IBR/Pi3 vaccines in calves less than 1 month old.

Other work has demonstrated that modified live virus BVDV vaccines provide protective immune responses to disease challenge when given to calves as young as 6 weeks of age. Little has been published regarding the effectiveness of vaccines against bacterial pneumonia pathogens such as Pasteurella multocida, Mannheimia hemolytica, or Mycoplasma bovis when administered to very young calves. Vaccine programs for calves against respiratory disease pathogens should be developed with advice from a veterinarian.

Detection of Respiratory Disease

To measure the success of the colostrum program, it is useful to have some benchmarks of calves morbidity and mortality. Less than

25 per cent of calves should be affected by disease (morbidity), and the death rate should be less than 5 per cent.

In order to evaluate the severity of the respiratory disease, some research suggests a respiratory score based on rectal temperature, the characteristics of the nasal discharge, eye or ear appearance, and presence of cough. The score is the sum of points from the four categories of clinical signs (temperature, cough, nasal discharge, eye or ear), where the higher the value indicates greater severity. Calves are considered sick when they score 6 or greater and present two or more clinical signs of respiratory disease.

Treatment and prevention

Once clinical signs of respiratory disease become evident in a calf, appropriate antibiotic therapy is warranted. Antibiotics will not affect viral infections; instead, antibiotics are directed against primary or secondary bacterial infections such as Pasteurella, Mannheimia, and Mycoplasma.

A wide variety of effective antibiotics are available, mostly as prescription drugs that may be obtained when a *valid veterinary client patient relationship* exists. Antibiotics typically considered effective against respiratory infections include tetracycline, florfenicol, ceftiofur, tulathromycin, and enrofloxacin, among others. Treatment is most effective soon after clinical signs are detected; medication failures are not uncommon when treatment is not initiated until late in the course of disease. Other supplemental treatments such as anti-inflammatory drugs may also be of benefit.

Treatment decisions should be made with veterinary input and with the use of diagnostic bacteriologic sensitivity results, if available.

Calf Scours

Calf scours seemed to be prominent in a number of herds during February and March of 2008. If you remember what our weather was like during this period, you will recall it was rainy and cool as cattle and cattleman alike battled mud and bone-chilling conditions. In fact, rain and mud lead to hypothermia, lower the calf's ability to resist infections, and can open the way for scours or diarrhea to occur.

There are a number of infectious agents that are responsible for diarrhea in calves, among them viruses and bacteria. The most common viruses associated with calf scours are rotavirus and corona virus. Both of these viruses infect and destroy the cells that line the intestinal tract. The calf looses the ability to digest and absorb milk. If the calf survives, this damage can be repaired but meanwhile the calf experiences serious fluid and electrolyte (generally potassium, sodium, chlorine and bicarbonate) loss from the accompanying diarrhea that leads to severe dehydration and acidosis.

The most common bacteria associated with calf scours/diarrhea is E. coli (Escherichia coli). This bacteria releases a toxin that damages the cells lining the gut, causing the normal absorptive capacity of the intestine to change and result in fluids and electrolytes being secreted and lost. This type of calf scours is generally seen only in very young calves up to about 5 days in age. There are also species of Salmonella bacteria associated with calf scours.

Under less severe cases of diarrhea or in early stages of diarrhea, calves exhibit loose stools, dryness of mouth and some loss of skin elasticity due to dehydration. More severe or prolonged diarrhea leads to worse dehydration and chemical imbalance in the body. Symptoms include: eyeballs beginning to sink into the eye sockets, calves become weak and lethargic, calves may be unable to stand, body temperature drops to below normal, and loss of nursing reflex. At this point, if calves are not treated they can move into coma, shock and then will die.

The most important treatment for calf scours/diarrhea is to replace the fluids and electrolytes that the body is losing. There are numerous commercial products available that can rehydrate the calf, correct pH imbalances and replace lost electrolytes. You may want to consult with your veterinarian as to a specific product and recommended volume/mixture to use in treatment of sick calves. A key point is to start fluid replacement early on while calves are still standing and have a nursing reflex.

If the calf will nurse from a bottle, electrolytes can be provided in this manner. If the calf refuses to nurse from a bottle, replacement fluids and electrolytes will have to be given by using an esophageal feeder probe/tube. Again, you may want to consult with your veterinarian about the proper use and placement of an esophageal tube. Keeping calves hydrated will help the calf to maintain vigour, enable the calf to continue to nurse, and help the calf to maintain its body temperature. Once a calf loses the ability to stand and suckle, the only recourse is intravenous (IV) treatment.

While antibiotics and sulfa drugs are commonly given as an oral treatment to calf scours, it has been found that this is not effective treatment and may even be detrimental. According to an article on calf scours by Don Hansen, Extension Veterinarian at Oregon State University, ". . . antibiotics and sulfa drugs given orally alter the normal population of organisms in the gut and sometimes predispose to super infections or fungal infections. Some antibiotics, when given orally, actually inhibit glucose absorption and alter the cells that line the gut wall. In these cases, continued oral use actually prolongs diarrhea."

Early fluid replacement treatment can be effective, but prevention of calf scours is, of course, preferable. Prevention goes back to management and understanding how scours can develop. Think of a triangle, with each leg of the triangle representing a factor that needs to be present for scours to develop. There are three: a susceptible animal, an infectious agent/organism and a favourable environment. Management practices that can reduce or break any of these legs of the triangle can reduce the severity of, or prevent scours from developing. A calf that is able to ingest a good quantity of colostrum, 5-6% of the calf's body weight within the first 6 hours after birth, is less susceptible to scours than a calf that nurses late or only ingests a small amount of colostrum. Vaccination programs that include an initial shot and a follow up booster to cows 6-7 weeks before calving boost antibody levels in the colostrum to provide added protection against early calf hood diarrhea/scours. Anything that can be done to keep the calf dry and relatively warm can go a long way in reducing a favourable environment for disease organisms and help to prevent occurrence of scours. Mud is the enemy in this regard.

Another management practice that should be followed as a preventative measure is to make sure that new replacement animals are NOT introduced into the herd within the two months prior to calving to two months after calving window. These animals could carry and introduce disease organisms that calves have no protection against from colostral antibodies.

Calf scours can be a disheartening experience during the calving season. Wet, muddy conditions increase the chance of calf scours. Anything the cattleman can do to provide warmer, drier conditions can help to prevent scours, along with making sure that a good first meal of colostrum is ingested soon after birth. Once scours develop, the most effective treatment is replacement of fluids and electrolytes.

Estrus Detection in Cattle

Heat detection is critical to heat synchronisation and breeding programs, particularly artificial insemination and embryo transfer programs. Effective heat detection is often the most limiting factor in an artificial insemination program. Heat detection can also be used to monitor onset of puberty in heifers, regularity of estrous cycles in breeding age females, and breeding effectiveness of natural service sires via returns to heat in the cow herd.

Heat detection efficiency (rate) is the percentage of eligible cows seen or detected in heat. Eligible cows are cows eligible for insemination. Heifers have reached puberty if they have resumed normal estrus function (cycling) after calving (typically 40 days or more postcalving), are free of reproductive disorders or reproductive tract infections, and are open. A heat detection rate of 80 to 85 per cent should be attainable.

Heat Signs and Detection Methods

Several methods of heat detection can be implemented. Some involve using heat detection aids. Several different methods can be combined to improve heat detection rates and accuracy. These include visual observation, heat mount detectors, tailhead markers (paint, chalk, crayon, paste), chin-ball markers, detector animals, and electronic heat detection devices.

Visual Observation

Visual observation is a commonly used method of heat detection. It involves a trained observer's recognising and recording signs of heat. Observable signs of heat include mounting or attempting to mount other cattle, standing to be mounted by other cattle, smelling other females, trailing other females, bellowing, depressed appetite, nervous and excitable behaviour, mud on hindquarters and sides of cattle, roughed up tail hair, vulva swelling and reddening, clear vaginal mucous discharge, and mucous smeared on rump.

The surest sign of heat is when a cow or heifer allows other cattle to mount her while she remains standing. This is called standing heat. Cattle may be willing to mount others but may not stand to be mounted when outside of standing heat. This usually indicates she is either coming into or going out of standing heat.

This method requires observation of cattle at least twice daily, typically early in the morning and late in the evening for best results. More frequent observation of cattle for heat improves detection accuracy and increases the likelihood of recognising the optimal time for breeding cattle, particularly in cattle in which heat is less intense or shorter in duration. Nearly 20 percent more cattle will be observed in heat when checked four times per day versus checking twice daily. Check cattle as often as practical. Space heat detection observation times evenly over 24 hours. Each observation period must be sufficiently long, usually at least 30 minutes, to be effective.

Standing heat can occur any time in a 24-hour period. However, the most likely time for a cow or heifer to show heat signs is at night. The season of the year can influence this, with more cows showing heat at night in hot weather and more showing heat during the day in cold weather. Housing conditions can also have an effect on the distribution of heat during a 24- hour period. Hot weather, high production, crowded conditions, and high stress environments may reduce mounting activity.

Observers must distinguish among cattle coming into heat, in standing heat, and going out of heat. Females that are in standing heat, were in standing heat yesterday, or will be in standing heat tomorrow are the most likely herd mates to mount other cows or heifers in heat. Observe cows away from the feed bunk so feeding behaviour does not interfere with heat detection. Cattle need nonslip footing and ample room to interact freely. Dirt footing increases mounting and standing activity more than concrete footing.

Heat Detection Aids

Heat detection aids are available. They should be used to supplement but not replace visual observation. These include tail paint, Kamar® Heatmount® Detectors, Estrotect™ Heat Detectors, Bovine Beacon®, tail head markers, chin-ball markers, and the HeatWatch® II System, an electronic detection system that records mounting behaviour. Heat detection aids differ in their application method, detection method, cost per animal, and detection accuracy.

Detector (teaser) animals can also assist in heat detection. Teaser animals include several types of gomer bulls, which are surgically altered to prevent successful insemination. Select gomer bulls that will not become excessively large. Acceptable disposition and freedom from disease are also important in gomer bulls.

Management Considerations

Good management is important for a successful heat detection program. Animals must have clearly readable, unique identification. An adequate area and equipment for heat detection must be available. This may include binoculars or the ability to approach cattle very closely. Nighttime observations may require artificial lighting, such as security lights, flashlights, or lanterns. Record keeping supplies such as paper, writing utensils, and clocks are important, along with a well-organised recordkeeping system.

Persons detecting heat must be well trained in heat detection and recording. Instruct all persons detecting heat to record cow or heifer ID, time of observation, and all signs of heat observed. Record all heat periods detected, even if the cow or heifer will not be bred on that heat. Then breeding wheels, calendars, or heat expectancy charts can be used to help predict future heats.

Summary

The effectiveness of detecting heat in cattle varies, depending on method used. Consider the cost, labour, and management system associated with each method in deciding on the best approach to heat detection. The purpose of heat detection also determines the level of heat detection accuracy needed.

Real-Time Ultrasound: Possible Uses in Genetic Prediction

By William Herring, Department of Animal Science, University of Missouri Extension. Ultrasound found its first applications in livestock research in the 1950s.

Since that time, the great strides that have been made in ultrasound research have benefited both human medicine and the livestock industry. Most people probably associate ultrasound with human fetal examination. In human medicine, it is most commonly used in routine pregnancy exams and sex determination. This same technology, including identical equipment, is used in the beef cattle industry to evaluate reproductive and carcass characteristics. However, this publication concentrates on the use of ultrasound to predict carcass merit, specifically genetic prediction for seedstock producers.

What is Ultrasound?

Technically, ultrasound is mechanical pressure waves, or sound waves, with frequencies above 20,000 hertz (oscillations per second). The portion of an ultrasound unit that actually emits and receives sound waves is known as a transducer. As sound waves are emitted from the transducer and pass through tissues with different densities, the echoes passed back to the transducer show this density change. For example, muscle and fat have different densities, thus allowing for their differentiation.

"Real-time" ultrasound is most commonly used in industry, although other ultrasound technologies are being investigated. Simply put, real-time ultrasound allows the operator to view the image while the measurement is being made. For example, when using real-time ultrasound in human pregnancy examinations, the heartbeat of an unborn child can be viewed on a television monitor.

Traits Measured

The most common traits measured in live beef cattle include 12-13th rib fat thickness, ribeye area, and percentage intramuscular fat. When measured in the carcass, 12-13th rib fat thickness and ribeye area are used to calculate U.S. Department of Agriculture yield grade. We also know that these two measurements, particularly fat thickness, account for an important amount of the variation in carcass cutability.

The trait having the most influence on USDA quality grade is marbling score. Although this is the most important commonly measured trait contributing to beef palatability, it accounts for only a small portion of the variation in beef palatability. Marbling score is an estimate of the amount of intramuscular fat present in the ribeye between the 12th and 13th ribs. Ultrasound can also be used to estimate the amount of intramuscular fat in the ribeye in live cattle. It is not an estimate of marbling score but a direct estimate of the amount of intramuscular fat present in the ribeye.

Accuracy, Precision and Repeatability

For ultrasound measurements to be useful in measuring fat thickness, ribeye area and percentage intramuscular fat, they must be accurate, precise and repeatable. Accuracy and precision are not necessarily the same thing. Think of precision as the ability of a technique to rank the measurements correctly. Accuracy would imply not only a correct ranking but also that the measurements taken were the same as some objective comparison. Therefore, measurements may be precise but not accurate.

For example, say the true average fat thickness on a group of fed steers is 0.6 inch, with the fattest being 1.2 and the leanest 0.2 inch. Ultrasound might rank the steers correctly but overestimate every animal by 0.5 inch. The ultrasound measurements might say the leanest steer was 0.7, the fattest at 1.7, with an average fat thickness of 1.1 inches. In other words, the differences between animals would be the same (1.7 - 0.7 = 1.0 and 1.2 - 0.2 = 1.0). These measurements would be precise but not accurate. If the ultrasound measurements were also accurate, the smallest ultrasound measurement would identify the lean steer at 0.2, the fat steer at 1.2 and the group average at 0.6 inch. For purposes of genetic prediction, contemporary groups of animals need only be ranked correctly. For predictions used to market fed cattle, measurements should also be accurate.

Useful measurements should also be repeatable. For example, if a group of cattle was measured ultrasonically one day, would the same measurement result if done the next day? If producers are using experienced, well-trained ultrasound technicians, the answer should be yes. For measuring backfat and ribeye area, research clearly indicates that when using qualified technicians, ultrasound can be a useful tool for gathering carcass information in live cattle. Recently, the Beef Improvement Federation has sponsored annual ultrasound certification programs. To be certified, technicians must pass accuracy, precision and repeatability tests for measuring 12-13th rib fat thickness and ribeye area and must also pass a written examination. A list of certified technicians is produced annually and can probably be obtained through your local MU Extension centre or your breed association office.

The prediction of percentage intramuscular fat is a newer developing aspect of ultrasound and has probably been the source of the most excitement. Several research groups across the country are working in this area. Early results are encouraging, but it is still unclear how useful this concept will be for measuring genetic merit in breeding animals.

Genetic Prediction for Carcass Merit

In the past and still for the most part, beef cattle producers are paid by the pound, whether it be for weaned calves, stockers or fed cattle at slaughter. Just as expected progeny differences (EPDs) have been used to alter growth, so can they be used to alter carcass merit. Studies from the University of Nebraska and the University of Georgia involving Angus-sired progeny indicate carcass EPDs do work and are valid means of altering carcass traits by selection. In the Nebraska study, six bulls with high marbling EPDs and six bulls with low marbling EPDs were bred to cows. In the Georgia study, nine high-marbling-EPD bulls that were below breed average for backfat EPDs and three control line bulls were selected for mating. Progeny were slaughtered and carcass data collected (Tables 1 and 2). Results indicate marbling can be increased while holding backfat at acceptable levels when using carcass EPD as the basis for sire selection.

Currently only a few breed associations calculate carcass EPDs. The main reason more associations are not calculating carcass EPDs is lack of, and difficulty in collecting, carcass data. Ultrasound may provide a new data source for calculation of carcass EPD.

Carcass EPD based on Carcass Data

Carcass EPDs produced to date have been based on slaughtered progeny data on sires of interest. Most of these data have been produced based on designed sire progeny tests. For purposes of EPD calculation, these progeny tests must be correctly designed to ensure correct contemporary group structure and sire connectedness across contemporary groups. These progeny tests may require producers to randomly mate a sire of interest along with other reference sires to a group of females from which the progeny will be reared in a single environment until slaughter.

These reference sires will most likely be bulls that already have carcass data from slaughtered progeny. For this kind of evaluation, you can see that artificial insemination, availability to large cow numbers, and ability to track progeny through slaughter are needed. From these data, traits that can be used include fat thickness, ribeye area, marbling score, hot carcass weight, USDA yield and quality grades, and percentage kidney, pelvic and heart fat.

While this is probably the most accurate method for calculating carcass EPDs, there are other disadvantages. Most seedstock producers do not have access to the large cow numbers needed. However, commercial bull customers that have the ability to do artificial insemination may provide a source of cow numbers. Let's say a purebred producer wants to collect carcass data on two of his young sires. This would require that these two bulls be randomly mated to a group of females along with at least one reference sire that already had progeny carcass data. For the sake of discussion let's assume a 50 percent conception rate from artificial insemination and a requirement of contemporary groups with at least 15 progeny by each sire of one sex. Assuming no mortality from conception to slaughter and a 1:1 sex ratio, 180 cows would be needed for this small test resulting in carcass data on 45 steers, 15 from each sire.

You can also see this is a time-consuming and possibly somewhat expensive process. Let's say it's not until a young herd sire prospect reaches yearling age that you decide to progeny test. Considering it would be a year later until resulting calves are born, another 14-18 months before they are slaughtered, a sire would be at least four and probably five years of age before that data could be collected and used for genetic evaluation purposes. However, in most situations, bulls are much older before owners decide to perform a progeny test. A more timely method of determining genetic merit for carcass traits is needed.

Though progeny testing requires a serious commitment on the part of the seedstock producer, it provides the only previously validated means of genetic prediction for carcass merit and cannot be overlooked by the serious breeder.

Collecting Ultrasound Data From Breeding Animals

Ultrasound may provide an opportunity to determine a sire's genetic merit for carcass traits much more quickly. Unlike actual carcass data, ultrasound provides a quick, nondestructive means of measuring the same traits in the live animal. Although there are still many uncertainties about when and how these measurements should be collected, several universities across the country are conducting research in this area.

What and When to Measure?

Unlike collecting slaughter data on commercial progeny, this approach involves measuring seedstock. More than likely, measurements would focus on young bulls. These groups of bulls would obviously include sons of herd sires but might also include other potential purebred herd sire prospects. So in a sense this approach is also a progeny test.

These measurements would more than likely be taken on groups of yearling bulls that had been developed on a higher-energy, post-weaning ration. On the average, bulls will not exhibit as much external or intramuscular fat as their steer counterparts. For purposes of genetic prediction, enough variation must be present to ensure that the animals can be correctly ranked.

At present, bulls should probably be measured using the same guidelines for collecting yearling weight that are used by your breed association (i.e., recommended yearling age ranges and contemporary group definitions within your breed association), although at this time there is no scientific basis for determining the optimum ranges. This will most likely be determined by the individual breed associations based on pending research results.

Growing heifers might also be measured. There is some concern over the future reproductive ramifications of feeding a group of growing heifers a ration that is sufficient for fat variation to be displayed. For females, it may be more appropriate to measure fat after a year of age, which would allow for more potential expression of external and intramuscular fat. Just as when considering traits such as birth or weaning weight, it is important that a contemporary group structure be defined.

A contemporary group is a management group of animals of the same sex that have had the same opportunity to perform. Anything that violates this definition, such as animals being reared in different pastures or being fed different rations, constitutes a separate contemporary group. For genetic evaluations, contemporary groups are necessary to remove effects of different environments and provide a means of analysing the genetic ties that exist between these groups. Therefore, accurate contemporary group definitions are a must.

However, just as with some of the other ultrasound areas, there is no research to indicate what contemporary group structure is appropriate. Can we group animals that were reared in separate pastures into single contemporary groups for ultrasound testing? More specifically, would those early environmental differences mask the genetic differences being measured ultrasonically? These answers are not yet available. When faced with variables of this type, it is in the association's best interest to use the most conservative contemporary group definition.

Who should take the ultrasound measurements? As previously mentioned, ultrasound technicians certified by the Beef Improvement Federation have been evaluated for accuracy, precision and repeatability. The cost of measurements may range from $10 to $20 per animal. Some producers in a single area may be able to coordinate with a single technician to reduce individual measurement costs.

Information collected would include an animal's tattoo, registration number, birth date and weight; ultrasound fat thickness, ribeye area and marbling; technician name; measurement date; and contemporary group.

Potential Concerns

From the standpoint of using ultrasound as a tool for gathering data for EPD calculation, there are still many questions that require further research. Most researchers would agree, however, that ultrasound is probably useful for genetic prediction of ribeye area. There is more concern with 12-13th rib fat thickness and intramuscular fat. More specifically, would ultrasound measurements for fat thickness and intramuscular fat on a contemporary group of bulls rank those animals the same if they were steers? Is it the same trait? Intuitively, we would say yes. Sex differences and the possible limited variation in those traits in bulls may lead to difficulty in genetic prediction methods.

Equipment, software and method of data collection are somewhat standardised for measuring 12-13th rib fat thickness and ribeye area with ultrasound. However, there are currently at least five different methods of measuring the percentage of intramuscular fat with ultrasound. The main differences occur with the software and algorithms used to analyse the ultrasound images. Some of these methods have undergone validation by the developers. However, it is unclear which of these techniques offers the most accuracy and would lead to measuring traits that result in the largest heritabilities.

Research is either currently under way or soon will be in all of these areas. Several breed associations are either currently collecting structured ultrasound data or have programs in place for collecting data.

Calculation of EPD

There is no doubt that ultrasound offers a potential means of calculating carcass EPDs for animals much sooner than the designed sire progeny test based on a carcass data. However, progeny tests based on slaughter data will still be useful. At least three different possibilities exist for the types of data used to calculate carcass EPDs. First, only carcass data based on the designed sire progeny test could be used. This is currently the only approach that has been validated by research. Second, a system using only ultrasound data based mainly on breeding animals might be used. Third, a system that would incorporate both ultrasound and carcass data could be developed. Even though the first method is the only one known to work, it will be in the best interest of the industry and research groups to make sure that the second and third options are successful. Most breed associations that do not already have carcass data collection programs in place, or breeders who have not taken part in collecting carcass data in those associations that do, are years away from a viable genetic prediction system. If the industry does shift to a true value-based marketing system, those groups that can provide their clientele with genetic information for carcass traits will be more competitive.

The Cascade and Human Generic Products

What is It?

The Cascade is a long-standing legal flexibility providing a rational balance between the legislative requirement for veterinary surgeons to prescribe and use authorised veterinary medicines where they are available, and the need for professional freedom to prescribe other products where they are not. It is intended to increase the range of medicines available for veterinary use.

Why is it Important to Use Authorised Medicines?

Animal species may have many physiological differences from humans and from each other. As a result they each may react differently to medicines. The authorisation system for veterinary medicines requires a product to have proven quality and effectiveness and, most importantly, safety for the animal, the user (vet, farmer, pet owner etc.), the environment and, for food animals, the consumer of animal produce. This assurance has to be provided for each species and each indication on the label.

In addition, animal medicines containing the same active ingredient as human medicines may be formulated differently. For instance, the formulation needs to ensure they are properly absorbed through the gut (which, for example, is rather shorter in a cat than a human). Human medicine formulations may contain different excipients or have different bioavailability from veterinary medicines. Using a product which is not authorised for animals therefore, increases the risk of harm to the patient.

In addition, the cost of developing a medicine for animal use is high and can involve much research and many tests not carried out for human medicines.

The use of human medicines, in place of the equivalent authorised veterinary medicine, can only be done by referring to the information on medicine use provided by the animal medicine companies. Assuming the data is transferable in this way is potentially hazardous and doing so takes advantage of work done by the animal medicine industry without paying for it. This means that those users abiding by the rules are subsidising those who do not, and such abuse diverts essential funding away from future research and development for new veterinary medicines.

It is important to address the potential confusion with the use of the word "generic". Authorised veterinary generics exist legitimately which can be used by vets as other authorised animal medicines. However, human generic medicines that are similar to the authorised veterinary medicines may not be used unless there is no suitable veterinary medicine available.

The Cascade provides a legal mechanism allowing veterinary surgeons to use their clinical judgement to prescribe a suitable medicine where no authorised medicine exists. Use and prescription by vets of human generic medicines where a suitable veterinary product is available is a criminal offence and contrary to the RCVS Guide to Professional Conduct.

Vets remain entirely responsible for the treatment of animals under their care; use of a medicine under the cascade should be capable of being supported by clear auditable clinical evidence to justify the vet's decision.

What Do Vets Need to Do to Comply with the Cascade?

If there is no medicine authorised in the UK for a specific condition, the veterinary surgeon responsible for treating the animal(s) may, in order to mitigate unacceptable suffering, treat the animal(s) in accordance with the following sequence:

(a) a veterinary medicine authorised in the UK for use in another animal species or for a different condition in the same species; or, if there is no such product;

(b) either:

　(i) a medicine authorised in the UK for human use, or

　(ii) in accordance with an import certificate from VMD, a veterinary medicine from another Member State; or, if there is no such product;

(c) a medicine prepared extemporaneously, by a vet, pharmacist or a person holding an appropriate manufacturer's authorisation.

If the animal(s) are food-producing animals, then the following additional conditions apply:

- the treatment in any particular case is restricted to animals on a single holding

- any medicine imported from another Member State must be authorised for use in a food-producing species in the other Member State

- the pharmacologically active substances contained in the medicine must have MRLs

- the prescribing vet must specify an appropriate withdrawal period – statutory minimums are in the Regulations

- the prescribing vet must keep specified records.

A medicine prescribed in accordance with the cascade may be administered by the prescribing vet or by a person acting under their direction. Responsibility for the prescription and use of the medicine remains with the prescribing veterinary surgeon.

Animals need medicines to help prevent disease and to help treat them if they do fall ill. All species deserve the benefit of medicinal products which have been specifically developed and authorised for their treatment. The cascade ensures this happens wherever possible, but also gives flexibility for veterinary surgeons to use their clinical judgement to prescribe a medicine where no veterinary authorised medicine exists

Consumer Attitudes to Animal Medicines

Introduction

In September 2006 the National Office of Animal Health commissioned the Institute of Grocery Distribution (IGD) to conduct research into consumer attitudes towards the use of animal medicines in farm animals. The key objectives were to:

- Explore consumer attitudes in the use of medicines and vaccination to treat and prevent disease.
- Establish the level of concern, if any, about the use of animal medicines.
- Understand the demand for information about animal medicines.
- Identify sources of consumer trust within the food chain.

Key Findings

The key findings were presented at the NOAH conference – "Healthy Animals Safe Food" in November 2006 and were:

- Animal medicines and vaccinations are not of great concern to consumers – main concerns are centred on hygiene in the factories and animal living conditions.
- Consumers have confused attitudes towards vaccination.
- The information most shoppers want is what feed animals receive (33%) and what hygiene standards exist (30%).
- There is a demand amongst 23% of respondents to know if animals have been fed or injected with anything to make them grow.

- The most trusted sources are independent bodies; the Food Standards Agency scored 29%. Other high scoring sources trusted for information include supermarkets and farmers.

Conclusion

Animal medicines and vaccinations are not of great concern to consumers, although three quarters claim to be aware of their use.

Demand for information is limited; reassurance rather than detail is needed.

Risk Assessment and Veterinary Medicines

Introduction

Along with every other business, those who hold a stock of animal medicines for sale or supply will need to carry out a COSHH risk assessment. But what does this mean in relation to animal medicines? Is a 'safety data sheet' needed for each animal medicine? And where can businesses get the information on medicines to undertake a risk assessment.

Advice from the Risk Assessments and the Veterinary Medicines Perspective

The RCVS publishes a which relates to risk assessments, states the following;

"The practice must have undertaken a thorough assessment of the risks arising from the use of veterinary medicines substances hazardous to health within the practice (L)"

The text goes on to explain how and why the risks posed by veterinary medicines should be assessed;

"The risk to Health & Safety from veterinary medicines and other substances has to be assessed under the Control Of Substances Hazardous to Health Regulations 2002 (COSHH).

There is wide variation in risk – many are low to medium risk but there are some substances in veterinary practice which pose a very serious risk to health.

Implementing measures to control the exposure to low or medium risk substances can be adequately achieved when they are assessed by their therapeutic group/type/route of administration etc. The practice can set out standard measures to control exposures, for example:

- Injectable anaesthetics;

- Pour-on anthelmintics;
- Steroidal compounds;
- Antibiotics.

Within these groups, practices must identify any specific medicines or substances that could have longer-term health risks, such as allergies e.g. Penicillin, or sensitivities e.g. latex

Specific and detailed assessments and the resulting measures to control exposure must be made for high-risk substances such as:

- Any hormones;
- Oil-based vaccines;
- Cytotoxic drugs;
- Gluteraldehyde disinfectants;
- Micotil (tilmicosin);
- Large animal Immobilon (etorphine);
- Zoonoses"

While this advice is aimed at veterinary practices, other businesses, such as animal health distributors and pet shops will also need to go through the risk assessment process.

In order to facilitate the risk assessment process, suppliers will need to have access to information about the veterinary medicinal products which they hold.

Do I Need a Safety Data Sheet?

The answer is, it depends, but the important thing to note is that a Safety Data Sheet is not required for every medicine.

In the eyes of the law, there is no such thing as a "COSHH data sheet." The correct term is "Safety Data Sheet" or "REACH safety data sheet."

REACH is a new European Regulation that covers the Registration, Evaluation, Authorisation and restriction of chemicals. It entered into force in 2007. REACH has replaced a number of pieces of older chemicals' legislation, including the Safety Data Sheet Directive.

Therefore, in the United Kingdom, the requirements for safety data sheets have moved from The Chemical (Hazard Information and Packaging for Supply) Regulations (CHIP Regulations) to REACH.

Veterinary (and human) medicines are exempt from some parts of REACH. In particular, medicinal products for veterinary use within the scope of Regulation (EC) No. 726/2004, Directive 2001/82/EC that are supplied in the finished state, intended for the final user are exempt from the requirement to supply a Safety Data Sheet.

Therefore, as long as the veterinary medicine is supplied in its final formulation and packaging for the final consumer, a Safety Data Sheet (SDS) is not required.

So, Safety Data Sheets are not legally required for veterinary medicines and many medicine companies do not produce them.

So How Can a Risk Assessment be Done?

Safety Data Sheets should not be confused with the Product Data Sheets and Summary of Product Characteristics (SPCs). Veterinary practices and other suppliers of animal medicines should ensure that they have access to the current version of either the SPC or the Data Sheet for each authorised medicine used or stored in the practice.

These provide all the necessary information to carry out the required risk assessment.

They are available in the current NOAH Compendium of Data Sheets and can also be found online at Alternatively, SPCs for all veterinary medicines can be found at:

SPCs for human medicines used by veterinary surgeons under the cascade (where there is no licensed veterinary medicine available) can be found at

It should be noted that the lists mentioned are not exhaustive and practices and other businesses stocking animal medicines should consider their own individual medicine/substance usage.

Veterinary Medicines in-use Shelf Life

What is an in-use Shelf-life?

An in-use shelf-life is the time period following the first broaching of a container (for example via a needle entering a bung or the unscrewing of a cap) after which any remaining product in the container should be destroyed. Veterinary medicines, human medicines, and increasingly other types of products such as cosmetics and shampoos specify an in-use shelf-life on their labels.

Why is it Necessary to have an in-use Shelf-life?

An in-use shelf-life is needed to provide assurance of the appropriate quality of the product throughout its use, thereby helping to ensure the safety and efficacy of the product. A product used outside its in-use shelf-life may have insufficient levels of the active substance and this may lead to inefficacy (or in some cases contribute to the development of resistance), or it may contain harmful levels of degradation products, or it may be contaminated with micro-organisms which would further challenge an animal whose health may already be compromised.

Why Don't All Medicines have an in-use Shelf-life?

Only products which are susceptible to degradation or contamination after first broaching of the pack carry an in-use shelf-life. For example, micro-organisms will not usually survive in non-aqueous environments. Therefore, for a non-aqueous pour-on product which has been shown not to be prone to degradation when exposed to the atmosphere an in-use shelf-life will not be specified.

Why Do So Many Medicines have a 28 Day in-use Shelf-life?

The in-use shelf-life specified depends on the product, in particular its physical, chemical and microbiological characteristics. The in-use shelf-life is not always 28 days. It may be less than this, for example if the active substance is prone to degradation following exposure to the atmosphere, or it may be longer than this, for example for a product which is very stable and which will not support the growth of micro-organisms (which can be the case for certain oily/non-aqueous injections).

However, many of the multi-dose parenteral (injectable) products do specify a 28 day maximum in-use shelf-life. The main reason for this is that the EU guidelines for veterinary and human medicines** on the "maximum shelf-life for sterile veterinary products after first opening or following reconstitution" both indicate that, from a microbiological point of view, for aqueous preserved sterile products and non-aqueous sterile products the in-use shelf-life should not normally exceed 28 days. There are examples of oily injections in the UK where the in-use shelf-life exceeds 28 days. In these instances the company has conducted additional microbial challenge studies beyond those set out in the European Pharmacopoeia.

Is it Possible to Extend an in-use Shelf-life?

Marketing Authorisation Holders (the companies who produce the product) can apply to the regulatory body who approve veterinary medicines, The Veterinary Medicines Directorate, in some circumstances to vary their authorisation to permit a longer in-use shelf-life. However, there will be significant additional costs involved in generating the data and significant costs involved in making the changes.

Another option to try to avoid wastage of medicines would be for Marketing Authorisation Holders to produce smaller pack sizes, but again this will involve varying the authorisation and is likely to involve the need for the generation of further data, with the inevitable additional costs that this involves.

In the past medicines where manufacturers had both large and small pack sizes on the market, a frequent problem that was encountered was that the smaller packs were not purchased and used by vets who were attempting to make savings based on economies of scale. As a result, the smaller pack sizes were discontinued.

Diagnosing Animal Diseases

Routine disease investigations are based on clinical, pathological and epidemiological evidence. If there is a need for conclusive identification of a disease or condition, an accurate laboratory diagnosis should be obtained. It is particularly important, especially in the case of infectious diseases that the final diagnosis rests on adequate aetiological evidence. In most cases disease investigations are carried out by qualified government stock inspectors and/or veterinarians. It helps for animal owners to understand and be able to recognise diseases conditions that may affect their animals, so that timely intervention can occur.

Course Structure

This course has nine lessons:

1. How Animal Diseases are Diagnosed - Conducting clinical examinations, gross and clinical pathology, information to collect and how to collect it (live animal and necropsy samples), specialist support services to assist in diagnosis (i.e. types of laboratories, specialist vets etc)

2. Diagnostic Testing - Pathways followed to detect and diagnose different types of diseases, information to be supplied with samples for diagnostic testing, and diagnostic techniques

3. Viral Diseases - Characteristics of viruses and the significance of a range of viral diseases that affect animals. You will study viral taxonomy, types and structure of viruses, virus replication cycle, transmission, and some common viral conditions.

4. Bacteria and Fungal Diseases - This lesson looks at the characteristics of bacterial and fungal organisms. Topics include: laboratory identification, controlling infections, specimen collection, and important disease conditions.

5. Parasitological Conditions - Discuss and differentiate a range of conditions that are caused by parasites. Topics include: Terminology and classification, life cycles, protozoa, helminths, and arthropods.

6. Metabolic and Nutritional Conditions - Lesson covers a range of common metabolic conditions affecting cattle, horses, pigs, sheep/goats, cats and dogs

7. Poisoning - Discuss and differentiate some common disorders that result from poisoning or toxins. These include: Cardio-respiratory, Central Nervous System (CNS), dermatological, gastrointestinal, hepatological, and haematological disorders.

8. Inherited Conditions (Genetic Disorders) - Discuss types of genetic inheritance, and give examples of genetic diseases affecting horses, dogs, and cats.

9. Other Conditions and Disorders - Identify and discuss miscellaneous conditions such as allergies, dehydration, and age related conditions.

10. Research Project -In this project you will evaluate symptoms of ill-health or disease displayed by a set of animals, and go through the process of identifying the problem and deciding on a course of treatment.

Extract from Course

Common Signs of an Ill or Injured Animal

The animal not eating as much as usual – this is usually the first sign you will notice. It may also drink more or less water than normal, depending on the illness. An animal standing by itself away from the herd Animal limping or dragging a leg Discharge from eyes, nose, or vaginal area

There may be abnormal lumps the eyes may be dull and the mucous membranes may have changed colour. Deep red membranes indicate fever; pale membranes show anaemia; yellow membranes indicate a liver disorder, while blue-red membranes show heart and circulatory problems, or pneumonia. Animal making unusual noise (bellowing, grunting)

Animal acting uncomfortable, getting up and down The animal might be sweating. A cold sweat indicates pain while a hot sweat indicates fever. If the animal is in pain it will probably be restless (getting up and down and pacing about), and it may even be groaning Diarrhoea or straining to defecate Animal not defecating or with very little stool Animal urinating a lot, or not as much as usual Marked weight loss or gain.

The coat will look dull and dry, and the hairs may stand up. There may the presence of open sores, dandruff, or the loss of hair or fur from the body behavioural signs - Recognise any significant differences in the behaviour of an animal such as increases in viciousness, lethargy or any other abnormal signs such as excessive head shaking, scratching, licking or biting of certain parts of the body. The vital signs of a sick animal will change. The temperature may go up or down. A rise in temperature of one or two degrees usually indicates pain, while a rise of more usually indicates infection.

The rate of respiration, and the way the animal breathes could also slow changes. With pain or infection, breathing becomes more rapid. In a very sick animal, breathing can be laboured and shallow. A slightly increased pulse rate suggests pain, while a rapid pulse suggests fever. An irregular pulse can indicate heart trouble. In a very sick animal, the pulse is weak and feeble. A sick animal may also possess foul breath or excessive tarter deposits on the

Understand How to Identify Animal Diseases

Improve your treatment of the animals you work with:

- Recognise problems before they become serious.
- Improve your business and/or career prospects.
- Taught and written by experts in the field..

Routine disease investigations are based on clinical, pathological and epidemiological evidence. If there is a need for conclusive identification of a disease or condition, an accurate laboratory diagnosis should be obtained. It is particularly important, especially in the case of infectious diseases that the final diagnosis rests on adequate aetiological evidence.

In most cases disease investigations are carried out by qualified government stock inspectors and/or veterinarians. It helps for animal owners to understand and be able to recognise diseases conditions that may affect their animals, so that timely intervention can occur.

Gum Disease in Dogs

Periodontal disease is an inflammation of some or all of a tooth's deep supporting structures. Today, it is one of the most common diseases in dogs.

If food particles and bacteria are allowed to accumulate along the dog's gumline, it can form plaque, which, when combined with saliva and minerals, will transform into calculus. This causes gum irritation and leads to an inflammatory condition called gingivitis. Gingivitis, which is evidenced by a reddening of the gums directly bordering the teeth, is considered to be an early stage of periodontal disease. After an extended period, the calculus builds up under the gum and separates it from the teeth. Spaces will form under the teeth, fostering bacterial growth. Once this happens, the dog has irreversible periodontal disease. This usually leads to bone loss, tissue destruction and pus formation in the cavities between the gum and teeth.

Periodontal disease affects both cats and dogs of all ages, though it is more common in older animals. If you would like to learn how this disease affects cats, please

Symptoms and Types

Periodontal disease generally begins with the inflammation of one tooth, which may progress if not treated during different stages of the condition. A dog with stage 1 periodontal disease in one or more of its teeth, for example, will exhibit gingivitis without any separation of the gum and tooth. Stage 2 is characterised by a 25 percent attachment loss, while stage 3 involves a 25 to 30 percent attachment loss. In stage 4, which is also called advanced periodontitis, there is more than a 50 percent attachment loss. In the most advanced stage of the disease, the gum tissue will usually recede and the roots of the teeth will be exposed.

Causes

Periodontal disease can be caused by a variety of factors. In dogs, the most common causes are the *Streptococcus* and *Actinomyces* bacteria. Canine toy breeds with crowded teeth, and dogs that groom themselves, carry a higher risk of acquiring the disease. In addition, poor nutrition will also contribute to the onset of the condition.

Diagnosis

The diagnosis of periodontal disease involves a number of procedures. If periodontal probing reveals more than two millimetres of distance between the gingivitis-affected gum and tooth, a dog is considered to have some form of periodontal abnormality.

X-rays are extremely important in diagnosing periodontal disease because up to 60 percent of the symptoms are hidden beneath the gum line. In the disease's early stages, radiographic imaging will reveal loss of density and sharpness of the root socket (alveolar) margin. In more advanced stages, it will reveal loss of bone support around the root of the affected tooth.

Treatment

The specific treatment for periodontal disease depends on how advanced the disease is. In the early stages, treatment is focused on controlling plaque and preventing attachment loss. This is achieved by daily brushing with animal safe toothpaste, professional cleansing, polishing, and the prescribed application of fluoride. In stage 2 or 3, the treatment involves the cleansing of the space between the gums and teeth and the application of antibiotic gel to rejuvenate periodontal tissues and decrease the size of the space. In the more advanced stages, bone replacement procedures, periodontal splinting, and guided tissue regeneration may become necessary.

Living and Management

Follow-up treatment for periodontal disease consists mostly of good dental care and weekly, quarterly, or half-yearly checks. Prognosis in dogs will depend on how advanced the disease is, but the best way to minimise the adverse affects caused by the disease is to get an early diagnosis, adequate treatment and proper therapy.

Prevention

The best prevention is to maintain good oral hygiene and to regularly brush and clean the dog's mouth and gums.

Bibliography

Alexander, D.: *Poultry Diseases,* Elsevier, 2007.

Allister, Mark Christopher: *Eco-man: New Perspectives on Masculinity and Nature,* University of Virginia Press, Charlottesville, 2004.

Archana Satarkar: *Food Science and Nutrition,* ABD Pub, Delhi, 2008.

Arora, N. : *Manual of Animal Nutrition,* International Book, 2004.

Aruna T. Kumar : *Handbook of Animal Husbandry,* Indian Council of Agricultural Research, 2008.

Balch M.D., J. and Balch C.N.C, P. : *Prescription for Nutritional Healing,* New York, U.S.A: Avery Publishing Group, 1997.

Baldick, Julian: *Animals and Shaman: Ancient Religions of Central Asia,* New York University Press, New York, 2000.

Balram Pani: *Textbook of Animal Chemistry,* I K International, Delhi, 2007.

Basu, T.K. : *About Mothers, Children, and Their Nutrition,* London, England: Thorsons Publishing, 1981.

Baudrillard: *The Animals: Territory and Metamorphoses. Simulacra and Simulation.* Ann Arbor: University of Michigan Press, 1994.

Benton, Ted: *Natural Relations: Ecology, Animal Rights and Social Justice,* Verso, London, 1993.

Betteridge, K.J. : *Embryo Transfer in Farm Animals,* Ottawa, Agriculture Canada, 1977.

Bhosale, Dinesh T. : *Handbook of Poultry Nutrition,* International Book, 2004.

Brock, J. : *A Natural History of Domesticated Animals,* Cambridge Univ. Pr., New York, 1999.

Brown, R. E.: *Social Odours in Animals Reproduction,* Clarendon Press, Oxford, 1985.

Budiansky, S.: *The Covenant of the Wild: Why Animals Chose Domestication,* Morrow, New York, 1992.

Chandra, Rajesh : *Diseases of Poultry and Their Control,* IBDCO, Delhi, 2001.

Clark, S. and S. Lyster: *Animals and Their Moral Standing,* Routledge, London, 1997.

Clark, Stephen: *The Moral Status of Animals.* Oxford: Oxford University Press, 1977.

Clymer, R. : *Nature's Healing Agents,* PA, U.S.A: Dorrance Co., 1963.

Coren, Stanley: *The Pawprints of History: Dogs and the Course of Human Events,* Free Press, New York, 2002.

Cox, N. A. : *Relationship Between Aerobic Bacteria, Salmonella, And Campylobacter on Broiler Carcasses,* Journal of Food Protection, 1997.

Crawford A. : *Experiments and Observations on Animal Heat,* London: Printed for J. Johnson; 1788.

DeGrazia, David: *Taking Animals Seriously: Mental Life and Moral Status,* Cambridge, New York, 1996.

Devender Pratap Singh : *A Handbook of Beekeeping,* Agrobios, 2006.

Dolins, Francine: *Attitudes to Animals: Views on Animal Welfare,* Cambridge University Press, Cambridge, 1999.

Donna Hill *: Biosecurity in the Poultry Industry,* International Book, 2006.

Edwards, L. : *Baking for Health,* New York, U.S.A: Avery Publishing Group, 1988.

Erasmus, U. : *Fats and Oils,* Vancouver: Alive Press, 1987.

Fairey, D.T., & Hampton, J.G. : *Forage Seed Production of Temperate Species,* Farnham Royal: CAB. 1997.

Flowerdew, J. R. : *Animals: Their Reproductive Biology and Population Ecology,* Cambridge Univ. Pr., New York, 1987.

Fox, Michael Allen: *The Case for Animal Experimentation,* University of California Press, Berkeley, CA, 1986.

Fraser, AF & Broom, DM.: *Farm Animal Behaviour and Welfare,* CABI, UK, 2004.

Gates, P.: *Animal Communication,* Cambridge University Press, Cambridge, 1997.

Guenter, W.: *Egg Nutrition and Biotechnology,* CABI Publishing, NY, 2000.

Hambidge, Gove : *Diseases and Parasites of Poultry,* Biotech Books, Delhi, 2004.

Harrison, R. J.: *Functional Anatomy of Marine Animals,* New York: Academic Press, 1974.

Homer O. Stuart: *Commercial Poultry Farming,* Biotech Books, Delhi, 2011.

Jacobson, M. : *Safe Food: Eating Wisely in a Risky World,* Washington, DC: Living Planet Press, 1991.

Katz, Jon: *The New Work of Dogs: Tending to Life, Love, and Family,* Villard, New York, 2003.

Keith Wilson N.D.P: *A Handbook of Poultry Practice*, Agrobios, Delhi, 2000.

Leclercq, B.: *Nutrition and Feeding of Poultry*, Nottingham University Press, U.K., 1994.

Mandal, A.B. : *Nutrition and Disease Management of Poultry*, International Book Distributing Co, Delhi, 2004.

Manning, Aubrey, and James Serpell: *Animals and Human Society,* Routledge, New York, 1994.

Mathialagan, P : *Textbook of Animal Husbandry and Livestock Extension,* International Book Distributing Co, Delhi, 2005.

McCollum EV. : *A history of nutrition,* Boston: Houghton Mifflin; 1957.

Moguilevsky, M. A. : *Drug Resistance of Enterobacteriacaea Isolated from Chicken Carcasses,* Journal of Food Protection, 1997.

Mohiuddin, S M : *Moulds and Mycotoxins in Poultry Diseases,* International Book, Delhi, 2007.

Morton, Eugene S.: *Animal Talk: Science and the Voices of Nature,* Random House, New York, 1992.

Nyholt, D.H. : *The Vitamin & Herb Guide,* Alberta, Canada: Global Health Ltd., 1992.

Owen, W Powell : *Poultry Farming and Keeping,* Biotech Books, Delhi, 2005.

Powell., C. : *Microbiological and Hydraulic Evaluation of Immersion Chilling for Poultry,* Journal of Food Protection, 1995.

Rakesh Kumar Shukla : *Handbook of Poultry Diseases : A Bedside-Guide,* International Book Dist, Delhi, 2006.

Randall, C.J.: *Color Atlas of Diseases and Disorders of the Domestic Fowl and Turkey,* Iowa State University Press, UK, 1991.

Raymond, F., Redman, P., & Waltham, R. : *Forage conservation and Feeding.* Ipswich: Farming Press, 1986.

Renaville, R and A Burny : *Biotechnology in Animal Husbandry,* Springer Pub, 2008.

Rifkin, Jeremy: *Beyond Beef: The Rise and Fall of the Cattle Culture,* Dutton, New York, 1992.

Rogers, Katherine: *The Cat and the Human Imagination,* The University of Michigan Press, Ann Arbor, 2001.

Sainsbury, D.: *Poultry Health and Management,* Blackwell Science, US, 2000.

Saxena, H.C. : *Poultry Feed Technology : Feed Formulation and Manufacturing,* International Book, Delhi, 2006.

Sharpe, Robert: *Science on Trial: The Human Cost of Animal Experiments*, Awareness Books, Sheffield, UK, 1994.

Short, R. V.: *Reproduction in Mammals*, Cambridge, Cambridge University Press, 1972.

Shukla, Rakesh Kumar : *Handbook of Animal Diseases : A Bedside-Guide*, International Book Dist, Delhi, 2006.

Singh, Ram Prakash : *Modern Livestock and Poultry Production*, Biotech Books, Delhi, 2008.

Snaydon, R.W. : *Managed Grasslands,* Amsterdam & London: Elsevier, 1987.

Tabor, Roger K.: *The Wild Life of the Domestic Cat,* Arrow Books, London, 1983.

Thornhill, Nancy W.: *The Natural History of Inbreeding and Outbreeding*, Chicago Press, 1993.

Thyagarajan, D. : *Diseases of Poultry*, Satish Serial pub, Delhi, 2011.

Ucko, Peter J. and G.W. Dimbleby: *The Domestication and Exploitation of Plants and Animals*, Aldine Publishing Company, Chicago, IL, 1969.

Watson, R.: *Eggs and Health Promotion,* Iowa State Press, UK, 2002.

Index

ooo